Advanced Osteopathic and Chiropractic Techniques for Manual Therapists

ADVANCED OSTEOPATHIC AND CHIROPRACTIC TECHNIQUES FOR MANUAL THERAPISTS

Adaptive Clinical Skills for Peripheral and Extremity Manipulation

Giles Gyer and Jimmy Michael

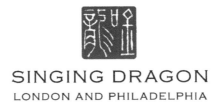

SINGING DRAGON
LONDON AND PHILADELPHIA

First published in 2020
by Singing Dragon
an imprint of Jessica Kingsley Publishers
73 Collier Street
London N1 9BE, UK
and
400 Market Street, Suite 400
Philadelphia, PA 19106, USA

www.singingdragon.com

Library of Congress Cataloging in Publication Data
A CIP catalog record for this book is available from the Library of Congress

British Library Cataloguing in Publication Data
A CIP catalogue record for this book is available from the British Library

ISBN 978 0 85701 394 1
eISBN 978 0 85701 395 8

Printed and bound in Great Britain

Contents

Disclaimer

To the fullest extent of the law, neither the Publisher nor the authors assume any liability for any injury and/or damage to persons or property incurred as a result of the instructions or ideas contained in the material herein.

This field is constantly evolving as new research and experience broadens our knowledge. As a result, changes in professional practice may be necessary. Therapists and researchers should rely on their own expertise in evaluating and using any information included in this book. They should be mindful of their own safety as well as the safety of others in their care.

With respect to any techniques identified, readers are advised to research the most current information available on procedures, dosage, method and duration of treatment, and contraindications. It is the responsibility of the therapist to provide the appropriate treatment for their patients, taking into account all the necessary safety precautions.

Over decades therapies have blended, and regardless of therapeutic title, we are all using to an extent similar techniques, just with differing philosophies. Spinal manipulation is utilised worldwide as an effective way to treat musculoskeletal pain and dysfunction. This book is merely to present effective techniques from our professions and should not be used unless readers have the relevant training and qualifications within manipulative therapy.

Acknowledgements

With special thanks to the following clinicians, whose help and contributions to this text have been invaluable:

Technique contributors

Dr Steffi Warnock, Master of Chiropractic (MChiro), Ireland

Dr James Inklebarger, MD, London, UK

Supporting contributors

Mr Chris Stankiewicz, BSc (Hons) Sports Therapy

Mr Rob Sanders, sports therapist

Images

Mr Adam Alex, photography (www.adamalex.com)

A special thanks also to Jacqueline Gyer and Anna Michael, without whose support this book would not have been possible.

1

SPINAL MANIPULATION THERAPY

Is it all about the brain? A current review of the neurophysiological effects of manipulation

Introduction

Spinal manipulation is a specialised form of manual therapy that uses non-invasive 'hands-on' treatment techniques to treat musculoskeletal pain and disability. The therapy has proven to be an effective treatment option for the management of various musculoskeletal disorders and is practised worldwide by health practitioners from various specialities, including osteopaths, chiropractors, naturopathic physicians and physiotherapists. However, little is yet understood about the physiological mechanisms of this therapy, especially how it exerts its pain-modulatory effects. Over the past decade, many theories have been proposed to explain the mechanisms of spinal manipulation (Evans 2002; Evans and Breen 2006; Maigne and Vautravers 2003; Potter, McCarthy and Oldham 2005), but the available data from mechanistic studies are insufficient to clarify the short- or long-term clinical outcomes of manipulation.

Most of the early theories that have been proposed to explain the analgesic and hypoalgesic effects of spinal manipulation were heavily focused on the biomechanical changes following the intervention (Evans 2002; Evans and Breen 2006; Potter *et al.* 2005). In recent years, however, there has been a paradigm shift towards a neurophysiological mechanism of spinal manipulation, as an increasing number of recent studies have reported various neural effects of spinal manipulation such as changes in somatosensory processing, muscle-reflexogenic responses, central motor excitability, motor neurone activity, Hoffmann reflex (H-reflex) responses, sympathetic activity and central sensitisation (Currie *et al.* 2016; Sampath *et al.* 2015; Lelic *et al.* 2016; Pickar 2002; Randoll *et al.* 2017; Zafereo and Deschenes 2015). These studies have suggested a cascade of neurochemical responses in the central and peripheral nervous system following spinal manipulation. Hence, it has been hypothesised that the observed pain-modulatory effects of spinal manipulation are largely due to neurophysiological mechanisms mediated by peripheral, spinal and supraspinal structures. These mechanisms have been thought to be triggered by mechanical stimulus or biomechanical forces applied during the manipulative act.

To date, Pickar's (2002) is the only review to provide a theoretical framework for the neurophysiological effects of spinal manipulation. Although Bialosky and colleagues (2009) later proposed a comprehensive model and a new framework to visualise potential individual mechanisms associated with pain reduction, their work was based on different forms of manual therapy and not exclusive to spinal manipulation alone. Hence, there has been a need for a comprehensive review that presents an updated framework based on the current knowledge and understanding of the neurophysiological effects of spinal manipulation. On the other hand, over the last decade a growing number of mechanistic studies have been conducted to understand the neurophysiological mechanisms of spinal manipulation. These studies have demonstrated various neural responses following manipulation. However, no review has been written to evaluate the relevance of these findings with regard to the proposed theories as well as the observed clinical effects. Therefore, the purpose of this chapter is to examine all the recent findings on the neurophysiological effects of spinal manipulation and review their relevance with respect to the improved clinical outcomes of spinal manipulation.

Discussion

Relationship between biomechanical changes and neurophysiological responses of a given spinal manipulation

The clinical effects of spinal manipulation are thought to be mediated by biomechanical and/or neurophysiological mechanisms. However, the exact mechanism(s) through which spinal manipulation exerts pain-modulatory effects, influences tissue repair and healing, and restores functional ability remains a mystery. Over the past decades, numerous hypotheses have been offered to explain these mechanisms, but evidence to support these theories is still limited. The evidence to date suggests that the effects of spinal manipulation are beyond biomechanical changes; in fact, a cascade of neurophysiological mechanisms may be initiated (Schmid et al. 2008). Biomechanical changes that occur due to spinal manipulation are thought to be produced by vertebral movement. The high-velocity, low-amplitude (HVLA) thrust introduced at the vertebral level during spinal manipulation mobilises the vertebrae on one another and is presumed to alter segmental biomechanics. In addition, the produced vertebral movement is known to be complex, as several adjacent vertebral levels are mobilised simultaneously (Maigne and Vautravers 2003; Potter et al. 2005).

There are four main theories of biomechanical changes elicited by spinal manipulation. These are (1) release of entrapped synovial folds or meniscoids; (2) restoration of buckled motion segments; (3) reduction of articular or periarticular adhesions; and (4) normalisation of 'hypertonic' muscle by reflexogenic effect (Evans and Breen 2006). However, the relevance of these theories on clinical outcomes remains uncertain. This is due to the fact that although a number of studies have quantified motion with spinal manipulation, biomechanical effects were found to be transient in nature (Colloca, Keller and Gunzburg 2004; Colloca *et al.* 2006; Coppieters and Butler 2008; Funabashi *et al.* 2016), and no plausible evidence has yet been found in support of a lasting positional change (Bialosky, George and Bishop 2008a). So far, only the muscular reflexogenic theory has some plausible evidence in support of its mechanical explanation (Clark *et al.* 2011; Colloca and Keller 2001; Currie *et al.* 2016); nevertheless, the clinical assertion that hypertonic muscles are influenced by an increased stretch reflex gain is not yet proven (Zedka *et al.* 1999). Furthermore, a common explanation widely propagated for the success of spinal manipulation is that it corrects changes in biomechanical dynamics, specifically position and movement faults, detected on examination. However, a majority of the current literature does not validate this explanation. This is because palpation has not been found to be a reliable method to identify areas requiring spinal manipulation (Seffinger *et al.* 2004; Walker *et al.* 2015), and the thrust applied during a therapy cannot be specific to an intended location (Frantzis *et al.* 2015) and varies between therapists (Cambridge *et al.* 2012).

The success of spinal manipulation in treating musculoskeletal disorders despite theoretical inconsistencies in its supposed biomechanical mechanisms indicates the possibility of concurrent additional mechanisms. Biomechanical changes evoked as a result of spinal manipulation may induce neurophysiological responses by influencing the inflow of sensory input to the central nervous system (Pickar 2002). Moreover, the mechanical force applied during spinal manipulation could either stimulate or silence mechanosensitive and nociceptive afferent fibres in paraspinal tissues, including skin, muscles, disc or discs, facet, tendons and ligaments (Currie *et al.* 2016; Randoll *et al.* 2017). These inputs have been thought to stimulate pain-processing mechanisms and other physiological systems connected to the nervous system (Bialosky *et al.* 2008a, 2009; Clark *et al.* 2011; Maigne and Vautravers 2003; Pickar 2002). In support of this hypothesis, Pickar and Bolton (2012) developed the notion that neural responses arising from the nervous system due to mechanical stimulus might be because of alterations in peripheral sensory input from paraspinal tissues.

Taken together, it can be said that changes in spinal biomechanics trigger the chain of neurophysiological responses responsible for the therapeutic outcomes associated with spinal manipulation, and there is a potential for combined biomechanical and neurophysiological effects following spinal manipulation. However, the possible interaction of these effects has frequently been overlooked in the current literature. The possibility of a combined effect is important to consider as biomechanical characteristics of a given spinal manipulation are shown to have a unique dose–response relationship with biomechanical, neuromuscular and neurophysiological responses (Cambridge *et al.* 2012; Downie, Vemulpad and Bull 2010; Nougarou *et al.* 2016). For example, paraspinal electromyographic (EMG) responses have an apparent dependence on the force/time characteristics of the mechanical thrust applied during spinal manipulation (Colloca *et al.* 2006). Therefore, future clinical studies should be conducted to investigate the relationship between variations in mechanical parameters (e.g., preload, peak force and thrust) and physiological responses and the relevance of varying parameters with biological and therapeutic outcomes.

Neurophysiological effects of spinal manipulation

Many authors have long postulated that spinal manipulation exerts its therapeutic effects by means of a number of neurophysiological mechanisms working on their own or in combination (Bialosky *et al.* 2008a, 2009; Pickar 2002). These mechanisms involve complex interactions between the peripheral nervous system and the central nervous system, and have been thought to be set in motion when spinal manipulation activates paraspinal sensory afferents (Pickar and Bolton 2012). The activation of sensory neurons is presumed to occur either during the manoeuvre itself and/or because of changes in spinal biomechanics. These paraspinal sensory inputs are assumed to alter neural integration either by directly influencing reflex activity and/or by affecting central neural integration within motor, nociceptive and possibly autonomic neuronal pools (Pickar 2002). However, since current biomechanical studies of spinal manipulation are unable to observe the changes occurring in the brain following the therapy – for example, how sensory afferent neurons produce neurophysiological effects by interacting with those in the central nervous system – the validity and relevance of theorised neurophysiological mechanisms in relation to therapeutic outcomes remains unclear. Implications for specific neural mechanisms of manipulation are suggested from associated neurophysiological responses, which have been observed in mechanistic studies.

Over the past decades, a number of specific and non-specific neural effects of spinal manipulation have been reported, including increased afferent discharge (Pickar and Bolton 2012), central motor excitability (Pickar 2002), alterations in pain processing (Lelic *et al.* 2016), reduction of temporal summation

(Randoll *et al.* 2017), stimulation of the autonomic nervous system (Sampath *et al.* 2015), lessening of pain perception (Bialosky *et al.* 2008b) and many more. These neural responses collectively implicate mechanisms mediated by the nervous system. Figure 1.1 presents a new theoretical model that illustrates the proposed neurophysiological effects of spinal manipulation based on the findings of current mechanistic literature. This model is heavily inspired by the comprehensive model presented by Bialosky and colleagues (2009), which was drawn interpreting the literature of several forms of manual therapy including nerve-based, mobilisation, manipulation and message therapies; hence, its relevance to spinal manipulation alone is unclear. The theoretical model we propose herein is diagrammed including only the literature on HVLA thrust manipulation.

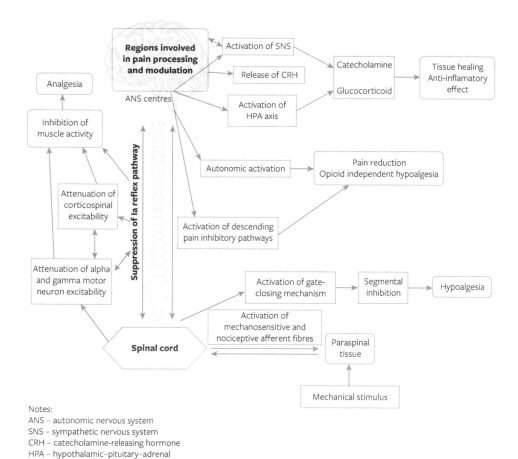

Notes:
ANS – autonomic nervous system
SNS – sympathetic nervous system
CRH – catecholamine-releasing hormone
HPA – hypothalamic–pituitary–adrenal

Figure 1.1. Neurophysiological and neurochemical effects of spinal manipulation

Neuromuscular effects

Muscle activation

The muscular reflexogenic response is an important theory that is frequently used to explain the mechanism of spinal manipulation. The muscles of the human body have some reflex responses, by means of their reflex arcs, to protect themselves from potentially harmful force (Evans 2002). In manual therapy literature, the reflexogenic effect is often explained using one of the prominent theories of pain, the pain–spasm–pain cycle (Travell, Rinzler and Herman 1942), which suggests that pain causes muscular hyperactivity (spasm) and muscle spasm reflexly produces pain, establishing a self-perpetuating cycle. Although this pain model lacks unequivocal support from the literature (van Dicĕn, Selen and Cholewicki 2003), there is enough evidence in support of the fact that low back pain (LBP) patients experience significantly higher levels of paraspinal muscle activity than normal healthy individuals during static postures (Geisser *et al.* 2004; Hodges and Moseley 2003; Lewis *et al.* 2012). Spinal manipulation is thought to disrupt the pain–spasm–pain cycle by reducing muscle activity through reflex pathways. Pickar (2002) postulated that the mechanical stimulus applied during manipulation on paraspinal tissues might influence the sensory receptors to cause muscle inhibition, and suggested that afferent stimuli would target this inhibition as a reflex response. Herzog (2000) proposed that the neuromuscular response to spinal manipulation could involve two reflex pathways – the capsule mechanoreceptor pathway and the muscle spindle pathway – and these pathways might differentiate by muscle activity onset delay.

EMG signals are commonly used to quantify changes in muscle activation following spinal manipulation. Amplitude and timing of the EMG signal are the two aspects that quantify muscle activity changes (Currie *et al.* 2016). Experimental studies done to assess neuromuscular responses to spinal manipulation reported both increases and decreases in EMG amplitude following manipulation (Bicalho *et al.* 2010; Ferreira, Ferreira and Hodges 2007; Lehman 2012; Lehman and McGill 2001). It is to be noted that most authors, including Lehman and McGill (2001), reported a reduction of paraspinal muscle activity following manipulation in resting phase. The conflicting results, however, appeared when EMG amplitudes were analysed during dynamic activity (flexion or extension). Nevertheless, most of the high-quality experiments published to date reported reduced paraspinal voluntary EMG amplitude during extension and relaxation phases (Lehman 2012). The changes in EMG amplitude in response to manipulation indicate that the underlying mechanism of spinal manipulation may involve the disruption of the pain–spasm–pain model.

The timing of the EMG signal is another measure of the muscle activity changes. Muscle activity onset delay quantifies the reflex response of a given spinal manipulation. Onset delay of a muscle following manipulation is too short, and varies in a wide range, from 1 to 400 milliseconds (Colloca, Keller and Gunzburg 2003; Currie *et al.* 2016; Keller, Colloca and Gunzburg 2003); thus, it is unlikely to be activated voluntarily (Herzog 2000). On the other hand, because a spinal reflex is assumed to take place within 120 milliseconds (Wilder *et al.* 1996), there is a high likelihood that a spinal reflex response may be involved with the muscle activity onset delay. Furthermore, in a recent study Currie *et al.* (2016) quantified differences in muscle activity onset delay between symptomatic and asymptomatic participants following lumbar manipulation, and found that those with LBP (symptomatic) had longer onset delays than their healthy (asymptomatic) counterparts, although the difference in timing was only 5 milliseconds. The authors suggested that the delayed neuromuscular response in the symptomatic group in response to spinal manipulation might be due to the involvement of capsule mechanoreceptor pathways. In support of this claim, they cited Herzog's (2000) work, where the author anticipated the faster activation of the muscle spindle pathways than capsular reflex pathways because of their reliance on large diameter Ia afferents.

From the above discussion, it is evident that spinal manipulation results in neuromuscular responses, involves spinal reflex pathways and may reduce muscle hyperactivity. However, it needs to be investigated whether the evoked short-latency changes in EMG amplitude and timing following manipulation indicate a clinically significant outcome or merely a short-term effect.

Modulation of gamma motor neuron activity

Korr's (1975) theory of the facilitated segment is a decades-old theory that has been used to interpret the mechanism of manipulation. From the early evidential basis, Korr hypothesised that a painful segment has a facilitatory response, and proposed that an increase in gamma motor neuron activity could lead to muscle hypertonicity by reflexly facilitating the alpha motor neuronal hyperexcitability. Korr suggested that spinal manipulation could calm the excited gamma motor neurons by increasing joint mobility, producing a barrage of proprioceptive afferent impulses. However, one major limitation of Korr's theory is that it lacked the neural pathways (i.e., afferent input likely to arise and reflex pathways that may be activated due to spinal manipulation) for its proposed mechanism of action. Interestingly, the pain–spasm–pain cycle (Travell *et al.* 1942) sheds some light on the possible neural pathway that may be involved in gamma motor neuron excitability. Johansson and Sojka (1991) proposed that this neural pathway would involve a hyperactive spinal stretch reflex, which is a process that involves skeletal muscle contraction and is thought to occur when the muscle spindles and Ia afferents are activated due to stretching of the muscle (Trompetto *et al.* 2014). Johansson and Sojka (1991) postulated that nociceptive afferents directly project on the gamma motor neurons, which react by increasing the output of muscle spindles, allowing the associated afferent nerves to signal changes in muscle length. This, in turn, results in the hyperexcitability of alpha motor neurons and subsequently leads to increased muscle activation.

As stated before, the pain–spasm–pain model is not unequivocally supported in the literature. Several authors have suggested that the sensitivity of muscle spindles is not affected by LBP, or paraspinal tissues do not undergo noxious stimulation (Birznieks, Burton and Macefield 2008; Zedka *et al.* 1999). Many studies still support the concept that spinal manipulation disrupts the pain–spasm–pain cycle and that it works by decreasing the hyperactivity of underlying nociceptors, consequently leading to stretch reflex attenuation and subsequent reduction in muscle activation (Herzog 2000; Pickar and Bolton 2012; Potter *et al.* 2005). Recently, however, two novel studies have established that with spinal manipulation, corticospinal or stretch reflex excitability can be attenuated. In the first study done to quantify the effects of spinal manipulation on stretch reflex excitability, Clark *et al.* (2011) observed an attenuation of stretch reflex of the erector spinae muscles when spinal manipulation produced an audible cracking sound. The authors suggested that manipulation might mechanistically act to reduce the output of muscle spindles and other segmental sites in the Ia reflex pathway. The second study was conducted by Fryer and Pearce (2012) on asymptomatic participants. The authors demonstrated a significant reduction in corticospinal and spinal reflex excitability following HVLAT manipulation that produced an audible cavitation. They also suggested that considerable alterations in corticospinal excitability could lead to changes in motor recruitment strategies.

These findings provide more insight into the possible segmental mechanisms of spinal manipulation. In addition, because an increased stretch reflex gain forms the basis of one of the neural pathways of the pain–spasm–pain cycle, it can be said that spinal manipulation may function via the pain model by attenuating stretch reflex hyperactivity, consequently reducing the hyperexcitability of gamma motor neurons.

Modulation of alpha motor neuron activity

The involvement of alpha motor neurons in the modulation of musculoskeletal pain has been proposed by two of the prominent theories of pain: (1) the pain–spasm–pain cycle (Cooperstein, Young and Haneline 2013) and (2) the pain-adaptation model (Lund *et al.* 1991). The pain–spasm–pain model proposes two distinct neural pathways that contribute to pain. However, both theories have one common basis: that hyperexcitability of the alpha motor neuron pool leads to increased muscle activity. One neural pathway is described above (see 'Modulation of gamma motor neuron activity'). Another pathway involves the projections of nociceptors onto alpha motor neurons via excitatory interneurons. On the other hand, the pain-adaptation model postulates that pain increases muscle activity when the muscle acts as antagonist and decreases it when active as agonist. The neural pathway proposed for this model involves feedback of nociceptive afferents projecting onto alpha motor neurons via both excitatory and inhibitory interneurons. The central nervous system (CNS) is thought to control the function of these interneurons and provide motor command of whether to excite or inhibit the alpha motor neuron pool (van Dieën *et al.* 2003). In short, regardless of the exact neural pathways, it may be said that the alpha motor neuron excitability forms the basis in the mechanism of musculoskeletal pain, as the modulation of alpha motor neurons correlates with changes in muscle activation.

Spinal manipulation has been thought to relax or normalise hypertonic muscle through modulating alpha motor neuron activity. However, the exact effect(s) of manipulation on motor neurons is still unknown. As described above (see 'Muscle activation'), most of the higher-quality EMG studies conducted to date demonstrated a significant attenuation of muscle activity following manipulation during forward bend or lying prone position (Lehman 2012). In a recent study on LBP patients, after observing reductions in EMG muscle activity during the flexion-relaxation phase, Bicalho *et al.* (2010) suggested that such decreases in EMG amplitude might be due to two different scenarios: (1) the hyperexcitability of the alpha motor neuron pool was decreased following spinal manipulation, or (2) manipulation increased the inhibition of the alpha motor unit. Nevertheless, the clinical relevance of EMG amplitude changes on the motor neuron pool is unclear, as EMG muscle activity changes were found to be transient in nature, and several studies have reported conflicting results.

Two experimental techniques that have been used to effectively measure motor neuron activity after mechanical stimulation include the H-reflex and transcranial magnetic stimulation (TMS). The H-reflex technique assesses the spinal reflex pathways that project onto the target muscle, bypassing the muscle spindle. It reveals an estimate of changes to the alpha motor neuron excitability following spinal manipulation (Burke 2016). In contrast, the TMS technique uses changing magnetic fields to measure the corticospinal tract excitability between the motor cortex and targeted muscle, evoking motor-evoked potential (MEP). It reveals the alterations in the motor cortex excitability after manipulation (Klomjai, Katz and Lackmy-Vallée 2015).

A series of studies conducted by Dishman and colleagues (Dishman and Bulbulian 2000, 2001; Dishman and Burke 2003; Dishman, Cunningham and Burke 2002; Dishman, Dougherty and Burke 2005) has consistently reported a significant but temporary attenuation of alpha motor neuron excitability after spinal manipulation using H-reflexes. One major shortcoming of these studies was that they lacked a no intervention control group. These findings, however, were contrasted by Suter, McMorland and Herzog (2005) who, after observing no alteration in H-reflexes in a subgroup, argued that the decreases in the H-reflex could be due to movement artifact during manipulation. In contrast, with a randomised controlled crossover design, Fryer and Pearce (2012) supported the findings of Dishman and colleagues but opposed Suter *et al.*'s (2005) conclusion. They reported that inhibition of H-reflexes was not associated with movement artifact as the control group showed no significant changes undergoing the same repositioning of the intervention group. More recently, in a cross-sectional study that included both asymptomatic healthy volunteers and subacute LBP patients, Dishman, Burke and Dougherty (2018) reported suppression of the Ia afferent-alpha motor neuron pathway and a valid and reliable attenuation of the Hmax/Mmax ratio[1] following spinal manipulation, which was beyond movement or position artifacts. This finding presents a completely meaningful physiological difference and provides convincing evidence in support of the long-held notion that HVLAT manipulation inhibits the excitability of the alpha motor neuron pool.

Since 2000, changes in MEPs following spinal manipulation have been examined by only a few researchers, and they reported conflicting results. While Dishman *et al.* (Dishman, Ball and Burke 2002; Dishman, Greco and Burke 2008) reported a transient but significant increase in MEPs compared with baseline after manipulation, Clark *et al.* (2011) found a slight decrease but no significant alteration in the erector spinae MEP amplitude. In contrast, Fryer and

---

1   An index for illustrating the level of reflex excitability of the motor pool, which, in turn, is dependent on the facilitation of the transmission between the Ia fibers and the AMN (alpha motor neuron).

Pearce (2012) observed a significant reduction in MEP amplitudes following manipulation. However, it is to be noted that Fryer and Pearce followed an established protocol to measure MEPs and recorded amplitudes roughly 10 minutes after the intervention, and thus speculated that a transient facilitation of MEPs might have occurred at the beginning. On the other hand, Dishman *et al.* observed that changes in MEPs returned to baseline 30–60 seconds following manipulation. Nevertheless, such conflicting data do not evidently indicate that spinal manipulation alters the corticospinal tract excitability.

Taken together, although spinal manipulation has been reported to result in a significant decrease in H-reflexes and EMG amplitudes, the clinical relevance of such short-lived changes on the motor neuron pool in the mechanisms that underlie the effectiveness of spinal manipulation is still speculative and needs to be determined.

Autonomic responses

The autonomic nervous system (ANS) acts largely unconsciously and controls the involuntary responses to maintain the internal body environment. It regulates several body processes (e.g., heart rate, respiratory rate, sweat and salivary secretion, blood pressure and pupillary response) and supplies various internal organs that have smooth muscle (e.g., heart, lungs, pupils, salivary glands, liver, kidneys, bladder and digestive glands). The system is regulated from the hypothalamus portion of the brain and is also in control of the underlying mechanisms during a fight-or-flight response (Cannon 1915). The ANS also has potential interaction with the nociceptive (pain) system on multiple levels, which include the brain stem, fore brain, periphery and dorsal horn (Benarroch 2006). Hence, any intervention that influences the functions of the ANS may have significant implications, as this may provide important mechanistic information and even shed some light on the possible neurophysiological mechanisms of that intervention.

In the manual therapy literature, autonomically mediated responses following spinal manipulation have been well established. A variety of outcome measures have been used to determine ANS activity after manipulation, including skin blood flow (SBF) indexes, blood pressure changes, pupillary reflex and heart rate variability (HRV). Studies performed to assess short-term changes in SBF following manipulation suggested a sympathoexcitatory effect, although this effect might be challenged because of overlooked local endothelial mechanisms regulating SBF (Zegarra-Parodi *et al.* 2015). Comparison of blood pressure changes pre and post manipulation has demonstrated ANS involvement (Welch and Boone 2008; Win *et al.* 2015). Pupillary reflex is also reported as an indicator of ANS activity (Sillevis *et al.* 2010). HRV is another well-established marker of cardiac autonomic neural activity, and reflects whether the sympathetic or parasympathetic branches of the ANS are influenced (Win *et al.* 2015). Therefore, it has been presumed that the effects of spinal manipulation on the ANS might lead to opioid-independent analgesia, influencing the reflex neural outputs on the segmental and extrasegmental levels (Sampath *et al.* 2015).

Significance of ANS changes following manipulation

Anatomically, the two complementary parts of the ANS include the sympathetic nervous system (SNS) and the parasympathetic nervous system (PNS). The interaction between both these systems is known to influence the stress response of tissues (Cramer and Darby 2013). The SNS plays an active role in mediating the fight-or-flight response and serves as a medium for the efferent communication between the immune system and the central nervous system. It releases catecholamine as an end product, which modulates several immune parameters during acute and chronic inflammation (Elenkov *et al.* 2000; Pongratz and Straub 2014). The mediating role of SNS between somatic and supportive processes has been demonstrated in Korr's pioneering work (Korr 2012). In addition, it has also been found that musculoskeletal abnormalities are associated with alterations in cutaneous patterns of sympathetic activity (Korr, Wright and Thomas 1962). In the manual therapy literature, this modulatory effect of the SNS on inflammation has been of special interest, as it may explain some of the neurophysiological effects observed after spinal manipulation. Hence, in the proposed physiological mechanisms of spinal manipulation, a prominent role of the peripheral sympathetic nervous system (PSNS) in the modulation of pain and inflammation has been theorised by both Pickar (2002) and Bialosky *et al.* (2009).

A number of studies since 2000 have investigated the effects of spinal manipulation on SNS changes. While some studies have reported immediate activation of the SNS following spinal manipulation (Budgell and Polus 2006; Welch and Boone 2008; Win *et al.* 2015; Zegarra-Parodi *et al.* 2015), others reported no change in sympathetic activity (Giles *et al.* 2013; Sillevis *et al.* 2010; Ward *et al.* 2013; Younes *et al.* 2017; Zhang *et al.* 2006). Welch and Boone (2008) suggested that the autonomic responses observed after manipulation might vary based on the specific segment(s) of the spine manipulated. The authors concluded that sympathetic responses are likely to be elicited from thoracic/ lumbar manipulation while parasympathetic responses might result from cervical spine manipulation. Several studies have supported this hypothesis to some extent (Budgell and Polus 2006; Giles *et al.* 2013; Win *et al.* 2015). However, contrary findings have also been reported. After measuring the HRV in healthy asymptomatic subjects at two separate time points, Zhang *et al.* (2006) reported a dominance of the PNS following thoracic manipulation. Recently, using both HRV and baroreflex sensitivity, another study (Ward *et al.* 2013) conducted on acute back pain patients has also demonstrated increased parasympathetic autonomic control after lumbar manipulation.

However, there were methodological differences between these studies, and no gold-standard technique was used to measure the SNS changes. In addition, the differences in findings were also somewhat dependent on the type of outcome measure used. It appears that the conflicting results mostly came from studies (Budgell and Polus 2006; Giles *et al.* 2013; Welch and Boone 2008; Ward *et al.* 2013; Win *et al.* 2015; Younes *et al.* 2017; Zhang *et al.* 2006) that used HRV analysis as a means to determine the nature of autonomic responses after manipulation. The findings of these studies were in favour of either the SNS or PNS. On the other hand, a recent systematic review on post-manipulation SBF changes has reported the presence of a short-term sympathetoexcitatory response (Zegarra-Parodi *et al.* 2015).

One possible reason for such differences might be the use of the low frequency (LF)/high frequency (HF) ratio as an indicator of ANS activity, where HF represents PNS efferent activity and LF corresponds to both PNS and SNS efferent activity. This method of assessing HRV has been criticised due to oversimplification of the complex non-linear interactions between the SNS and PNS (Billman 2013). More recently, Sampath *et al.* (2017), using a reliable measure (near-infrared spectroscopy) to assess SNS activity, reported an immediate sympathetic excitation following thoracic manipulation. Interestingly, this study also investigated pre and post manipulation HRV data but found no statistically significant difference between the groups. Nevertheless, the findings of this study need to be interpreted cautiously, as it was based on asymptomatic male subjects, and there has been a report of ANS dysregulation in chronic pain patients. Hence, more research on symptomatic population is warranted.

Effects of manipulation-induced autonomic changes on supraspinal mechanisms

As discussed above, there is a complex interaction between the ANS and the pain system, and the PSNS plays a significant role in modulating pain and inflammation. Hence, considering the evidence of immediate sympathetoexcitatory responses following manipulation, Sampath *et al.* (2015) suggested that these SNS changes might be linked to changes in pain-modulating supraspinal mechanisms. In support of this hypothesis, the authors cited two imaging studies (Ogura *et al.* 2011; Sparks *et al.* 2013) that demonstrated the effects of manipulation on several supraspinal structures including the cerebellar vermis, middle temporal gyrus, insular cortex, inferior prefrontal cortex and anterior cingulate cortex. All these structures have been reported to be involved in the regulation of autonomic function (Kenney and Ganta 2011). On the other hand, there has been a growing body of evidence in support of the manipulation-induced neural plastic changes (Daligadu *et al.* 2013; Lelic *et al.* 2016; Taylor and Murphy 2010) occurring in various brain structures such as the cerebellum, basal ganglia, prefrontal cortex, primary sensory cortex and primary motor cortex. Taken together, although there is no direct evidence in support of Sampath *et al.*'s (2015) hypothesis, this might be a fruitful area of research for future studies.

Co-activation of the neuroendocrine system

The hypothalamus region is known for coordinating stress responses by activating the hypothalamic–pituitary (HP) axis and a neural pathway involving the PSNS. The hypothalamic–pituitary–adrenal (HPA) axis has been considered to be the central stress response system and is known to release adrenal glucocorticoid (cortisol), which is a class of corticosteroids that are well recognised in the literature for their anti-inflammatory and immunosuppressive actions (Ulrich-Lai and Herman 2009). On the other hand, as discussed above, the SNS has been reported to serve as a mediator between the somatic and supportive processes. Hence, it has been well established that both the SNS and HPA axis could play a significant role in the modulation of acute and chronic inflammation, and the neuroendocrine (SNS–HPA axis) mechanisms are involved in the pain relief and tissue-healing processes (Chrousos 2009; Ulrich-Lai and Herman 2009). These two systems have also been reported to work together, overlapping the underlying neural circuitry (Chrousos 2009). In addition, the evidence suggests that spinal manipulation could influence the activity of both the SNS and HPA axis. Several studies have assessed the effect of spinal manipulation on the HPA axis, and an immediate increase in serum cortisol levels following manipulation has been observed in both symptomatic and asymptomatic patients (Padayachy *et al.* 2010; Plaza-Manzano *et al.* 2014).

Considering the above facts, Sampath *et al.* (2015) hypothesised that there could be an association between SNS changes and HPA axis responses, and post-manipulation changes in the SNS might be accompanied by HPA axis changes. The authors proposed possible neural reflex pathways in support of this hypothesis. They suggested that HVLAT at the thoracolumbar segment of the spine would result in excitation of the preganglionic sympathetic cells and subsequent stimulation of mechanoreceptors. These inputs would then travel to several regions of the brain stem and subsequently would lead to opioid-independent analgesia by influencing the hypothalamus and PAG (periaqueductal grey) matter in the midbrain. The hypothalamic release of the corticotropin-releasing factor (CRF) would then occur to modulate the SNS and HPA axis response. The neuroendocrine (SNS–HPA axis) system would then release its end products (catecholamines and glucocorticoids) to initiate anti-inflammatory and tissue-healing actions. However, to date, only one study (Sampath *et al.* 2017) has been conducted to investigate the SNS–HPA axis response to manipulation in the same trial. Although this study reported a reduction in salivary cortisol level immediately after thoracic manipulation and observed an immediate effect of manipulation on the SNS, the clinical relevance of such changes is so far unknown. Therefore, more research is needed to determine the true clinical significance of neuroendocrine response following manipulation.

Hypoalgesic effects

It is thought that four types of mechanism contribute to the hypoalgesic effects of spinal manipulation.

Segmental inhibition

The concept of this mechanism is based on Melzack and Wall's (1965) gate control theory of pain. This theory proposes that nociceptive (small diameter) A-delta (A-δ) and C sensory fibres carry the pain stimuli to the dorsal horn and 'open' the substantia gelatinosa layer, whereas non-nociceptive (large diameter) A-β fibres inhibit the transmission of pain signals by blocking the entry of A-δ and C fibres. Because mechanical stimulus applied during spinal manipulation may alter peripheral sensory input from paraspinal tissues, it has been presumed that manipulation may influence the gate-closing mechanism by stimulating the A-β fibres from muscle spindles and facet joint mechanoreceptors (Potter *et al.* 2005). Systematic reviews by Millan *et al.* (2012) and Coronado *et al.* (2012) have critically reviewed studies that examined the hypoalgesic effects of spinal manipulation on experimentally induced pain. Most of the studies included in these two reviews observed a segmental hypoalgesic effect of manipulation, and suggested that supraspinal pathways might be involved in the segmental mechanism. In addition, the involvement of a segmental mechanism in the modulation of pain perception has also been proposed by numerous studies investigating the neuromuscular effects of spinal manipulation (see 'Neuromuscular effects'). However, it needs to be determined whether the observed local hypoalgesic effect following manipulation is merely a reflex effect on the pre-existing painful condition itself or due to activation of the endogenous pain inhibitory system.

Activation of descending pain inhibitory pathways

This mechanism is based on the effects of spinal manipulation on the pain-modulatory neural circuitry. Manipulation has long been thought to modulate the non-opioid hypoalgesic system by activating the descending pain-modulation circuit, especially serotonin and noradrenaline pathways, from the PAG and rostral ventromedial medulla (RVM) of the brain stem (Pickar 2002; Vernon 2000; Wright 1995). This hypothesis has been supported by both animal model and human studies. In laboratory animal models (Reed *et al.* 2014; Skyba *et al.* 2003; Song *et al.* 2006), objective evidence has been found in support of a central antinociceptive effect that appeared to be mediated by serotoninergic and noradrenergic inhibitory pathways. The findings of human studies (Alonso-Perez *et al.* 2017; O'Neill, Ødegaard-Olsen and Søvde 2015; Sterling, Jull and Wright 2001) conducted on both symptomatic and asymptomatic subjects are also consistent with the findings of animal models. However, although human research supports a non-opioid form of manipulation-induced hypoalgesic effect through activation of some type of descending inhibitory mechanism, the exact circuit is yet not agreed upon. Because neural responses following spinal manipulation may vary depending on the rate of force application and the location at which the thrust is applied (Cambridge *et al.* 2012; Downie *et al.* 2010; Nougarou *et al.* 2016), it has been assumed that variations in mechanical parameters of manipulation may activate different descending inhibitory pathways (Savva, Giakas and Efstathiou 2014). Therefore, future research should be performed to investigate the exact descending pain-modulatory circuit involved after spinal manipulation, and these studies should also carefully consider the force/time and contact site characteristics of the given intervention.

Non-specific cerebral responses

The relevance of non-specific variables such as expectation and psychosocial factors in the mechanisms of spinal manipulation cannot be totally dismissed (Bialosky et al. 2009). Expectation of good functional outcomes may decrease pain perception without spinal involvement. In addition, a systematic review indicated that spinal manipulation is associated with better psychological outcomes than verbal interventions (Williams et al. 2007). However, studies done to determine the influence of non-specific cerebral processes in manipulation-induced hypoalgesia have found that manipulation has greater and specific effects on pain sensitivity than expectations of receiving the intervention (Bialosky et al. 2008b, 2014). Nevertheless, additional work is needed to determine whether application of spinal manipulation with increased positive expectations could provide an additive effect on pain perception.

Temporal summation

The effects of spinal manipulation on temporal summation of pain constitutes another experimental model that can be used to explain the mechanisms of manipulation-induced hypoalgesia. Temporal summation refers to an increased perception of pain evoked by repetitive painful (noxious) stimulus of the same amplitude and frequency. It represents a psychophysical correlate of a frequency-dependent, progressively increasing excitability of dorsal horn neurons (i.e., wind-up) (Anderson et al. 2013). Wind-up is an interesting model to study for manual therapy researchers, as it is a central phenomenon and not mediated by peripheral mechanisms (Herrero, Laird and Lopez-Garcia 2000). The constant nociceptive input into dorsal horn neurons through temporal summation can trigger transcriptional and translational changes that are related to the short-lived aspect of central sensitisation (Anderson et al. 2013; Staud et al. 2007). Thus, temporal summation can be used to characterise mechanisms of central processing in chronic pain conditions.

Early experimental studies (Bialosky *et al.* 2008b; George *et al.* 2006) done with cutaneous heat application to examine the effects of lumbar spinal manipulation reported immediate reduction of temporal summation in the lower extremity regions but not in upper limb dermatomes. This finding suggested that the hypoalgesic effects observed following manipulation might be regionally specific or segmental in nature. To confirm this hypothesis, Bishop, Beneciuk and George (2011) conducted a study to test whether thoracic spinal manipulation reduces temporal summation of pain. In contrast to earlier findings, they found that temporal summation was reduced in both upper and lower extremities, which suggested an involvement of both segmental and descending inhibitory mechanisms in manipulation-induced hypoalgesia. Recently, Randoll *et al.* (2017), using repeated electrical stimulus, also found that temporal summation of pain was reduced by thoracic spinal manipulation. The authors supported an involvement of segmental mechanism and suggested that deep high-threshold mechanoreceptors might be responsible for HVLA-induced hypoalgesia. However, further research is needed to establish the clinical relevance of these findings.

Conclusion

In this study, we discussed various theories proposed to date to explain the neurophysiological effects of spinal manipulation, and reviewed the mechanistic studies that have been done to validate the relevance of these theories. So far, the exact mechanism(s) through which spinal manipulation works has not been established. Experimental models conducted on both animal and human subjects have indicated that mechanical stimulus applied during manipulation produces a barrage of input into the dorsal horn of the spinal cord, which initiates a cascade of neural responses involving complex interactions between the PNS and CNS. Observing neurophysiological responses following spinal manipulation, these models have suggested possible mechanisms underlying the neuromuscular, autonomic, neuroendocrine and hypoalgesic effects of manipulation. However, the relevance of these implications in relation to the observed clinical effects remains unclear. This is because a majority of the mechanistic studies published to date have mainly investigated short-latency changes or immediate effects of spinal manipulation using their experimental models. In addition, the dose–response relationship associated with the specific neural effect of manipulation has frequently been overlooked in the current literature. Therefore, future studies projected at understanding the possible neural mechanisms of spinal manipulation should carefully consider these two variables.

References

Alonso-Perez, J.L., Lopez-Lopez, A., La Touche, R., Lerma-Lara, S., Suarez, E., Rojas, J. et al. (2017) 'Hypoalgesic effects of three different manual therapy techniques on cervical spine and psychological interaction: A randomized clinical trial.' *Journal of Bodywork and Movement Therapies* 21(4), 798–803. Available at www.ncbi.nlm.nih.gov/pubmed/29037630

Anderson, R.J., Craggs, J.G., Bialosky, J.E., Bishop, M.D., George, S.Z., Staud, R. et al. (2013) 'Temporal summation of second pain: Variability in responses to a fixed protocol.' *European Journal of Pain* 17(1), 67–74. Available at www.ncbi.nlm.nih.gov/pubmed/22899549

Benarroch, E.E. (2006) 'Pain-autonomic interactions.' *Neurological Sciences* 27(Suppl. 2), S130–S133. Available at www.ncbi.nlm.nih.gov/pubmed/16688616

Bialosky, J.E., George, S.Z. and Bishop, M.D. (2008a) 'How spinal manipulative therapy works: Why ask why?' *Journal of Orthopaedic & Sports Physical Therapy* 38(6), 293–295. Available at www.ncbi.nlm.nih.gov/pubmed/18515964

Bialosky, J.E., Bishop, M.D., Price, D.D., Robinson, M.E. and George, S.Z. (2009) 'The mechanisms of manual therapy in the treatment of musculoskeletal pain: A comprehensive model.' *Manual Therapy* 14(5), 531–538. Available at www.ncbi.nlm.nih.gov/pubmed/19027342

Bialosky, J.E., Bishop, M.D., Robinson, M.E., Barabas, J.A. and George, S.Z. (2008b) 'The influence of expectation on spinal manipulation induced hypoalgesia: An experimental study in normal subjects.' *BMC Musculoskeletal Disorders* 9(1), 19. Available at www.ncbi.nlm.nih.gov/pubmed/18267029

Bialosky, J.E., George, S.Z., Horn, M.E., Price, D.D., Staud, R. and Robinson, M.E. (2014) 'Spinal manipulative therapy – Specific changes in pain sensitivity in individuals with low back pain (NCT01168999).' *The Journal of Pain* 15(2), 136–148. Available at www.ncbi.nlm.nih.gov/pubmed/24361109

Bicalho, E., Setti, J.A., Macagnan, J., Cano, J.L. and Manffra, E.F. (2010) 'Immediate effects of a high-velocity spine manipulation in paraspinal muscles activity of nonspecific chronic low-back pain subjects.' *Manual Therapy* 15(5), 469–475. Available at www.ncbi.nlm.nih.gov/pubmed/20447857

Billman, G.E. (2013) 'The effect of heart rate on the heart rate variability response to autonomic interventions.' *Frontiers in Physiology* 4, 222. Available at www.ncbi.nlm.nih.gov/pubmed/23986716

Birznieks, I., Burton, A.R. and Macefield, V.G. (2008) 'The effects of experimental muscle and skin pain on the static stretch sensitivity of human muscle spindles in relaxed leg muscles.' *Journal of Physiology* 586(11), 2713–2723. Available at www.ncbi.nlm.nih.gov/pubmed/18403422

Bishop, M.D., Beneciuk, J.M. and George, S.Z. (2011) 'Immediate reduction in temporal sensory summation after thoracic spinal manipulation.' *The Spine Journal* 11(5), 440–446. Available at www.ncbi.nlm.nih.gov/pubmed/21463970

Budgell, B. and Polus, B. (2006) 'The effects of thoracic manipulation on heart rate variability: A controlled crossover trial.' *Journal of Manipulative and Physiological Therapeutics* 29(8), 603–610. Available at www.ncbi.nlm.nih.gov/pubmed/17045093

Burke, D. (2016) 'Clinical uses of H reflexes of upper and lower limb muscles.' *Clinical Neurophysiology Practice* 1, 9–17. Available at www.ncbi.nlm.nih.gov/pubmed/30214954

Cambridge, E.D., Triano, J.J., Ross, J.K. and Abbott, M.S. (2012) 'Comparison of force development strategies of spinal manipulation used for thoracic pain.' *Manual Therapy* 17(3), 241–245. Available at www.ncbi.nlm.nih.gov/pubmed/22386279

Cannon, W.B. (1915) *Bodily Changes in Pain, Hunger, Fear, and Rage: An Account of Recent Researches into the Function of Emotional Excitement.* New York: Cornell University Library.

Chrousos, G.P. (2009) 'Stress and disorders of the stress system.' *Nature Reviews Endocrinology* 5(7), 374–381. Available at www.ncbi.nlm.nih.gov/pubmed/19488073

Clark, B.C., Goss, D.A. Jr, Walkowski, S., Hoffman, R.L., Ross, A. and Thomas, J.S. (2011) 'Neurophysiologic effects of spinal manipulation in patients with chronic low back pain.' *BMC Musculoskeletal Disorders* 12(1), 170. Available at www.ncbi.nlm.nih.gov/pubmed/21781310

Colloca, C.J. and Keller, T.S. (2001) 'Stiffness and neuromuscular reflex response of the human spine to posteroanterior manipulative thrusts in patients with low back pain.' *Journal of Manipulative and Physiological Therapeutics* 24(8), 489–500. Available at www.ncbi.nlm.nih.gov/pubmed/11677547

Colloca, C.J., Keller, T.S. and Gunzburg, R. (2003) 'Neuromechanical characterization of in vivo lumbar spinal manipulation. Part II. Neurophysiological response.' *Journal of Manipulative and Physiological Therapeutics* 26(9), 579–591. Available at www.ncbi.nlm.nih.gov/pubmed/14673407

Colloca, C.J., Keller, T.S. and Gunzburg, R. (2004) 'Biomechanical and neurophysiological responses to spinal manipulation in patients with lumbar radiculopathy.' *Journal of Manipulative and Physiological Therapeutics* 27(1), 1–15. Available at www.ncbi.nlm.nih.gov/pubmed/14739869

Colloca, C.J., Keller, T.S., Harrison, D.E., Moore, R.J., Gunzburg, R. and Harrison, D.D. (2006) 'Spinal manipulation force and duration affect vertebral movement and neuromuscular responses.' *Clinical Biomechanics* 21(3), 254–262. Available at www.ncbi.nlm.nih.gov/pubmed/16378668

Cooperstein, R., Young, M. and Haneline, M. (2013) 'Interexaminer reliability of cervical motion palpation using continuous measures and rater confidence levels.' *The Journal of the Canadian Chiropractic Association* 57(2), 156–164. www.ncbi.nlm.nih.gov/pubmed/23754861

Coppieters, M.W. and Butler, D.S. (2008) 'Do "sliders" slide and "tensioners" tension? An analysis of neurodynamic techniques and considerations regarding their application.' *Manual Therapy* 13(3), 213–221. Available at www.ncbi.nlm.nih.gov/pubmed/17398140

Coronado, R.A., Gay, C.W., Bialosky, J.E., Carnaby, G.D., Bishop, M.D. and George, S.Z. (2012) 'Changes in pain sensitivity following spinal manipulation: A systematic review and meta-analysis.' *Journal of Electromyography and Kinesiology* 22(5), 752–767. Available at www.ncbi.nlm.nih.gov/pubmed/22296867

Cramer, G. and Darby, S. (2013) *Clinical Anatomy of the Spine, Spinal Cord, and ANS.* 3rd edn. Maryland Heights, MI: Mosby. Available at www.elsevier.com/books/clinical-anatomy-of-the-spine-spinal-cord-and-ans/9780323079549

Currie, S.J., Myers, C.A., Durso, C., Enebo, B.A. and Davidson, B.S. (2016) 'The neuromuscular response to spinal manipulation in the presence of pain.' *Journal of Manipulative and Physiological Therapeutics* 39(4), 288–293. Available at www.ncbi.nlm.nih.gov/pubmed/27059250

Daligadu, J., Haavik, H., Yielder, P.C., Baarbe, J. and Murphy, B. (2013) 'Alterations in cortical and cerebellar motor processing in subclinical neck pain patients following spinal manipulation.' *Journal of Manipulative and Physiological Therapeutics* 36(8), 527–537. Available at www.ncbi.nlm.nih.gov/pubmed/24035521

Dishman, J.D. and Bulbulian, R. (2000) 'Spinal reflex attenuation associated with spinal manipulation.' *Spine* 25(19), 2519–2524. Available at www.ncbi.nlm.nih.gov/pubmed/11013505

Dishman, J.D. and Bulbulian, R. (2001) 'Comparison of effects of spinal manipulation and massage on motoneuron excitability.' *Electromyography and Clinical Neurophysiology* 41(2), 97–106. Available at www.ncbi.nlm.nih.gov/pubmed/11284061

Dishman, J.D. and Burke, J. (2003) 'Spinal reflex excitability changes after cervical and lumbar spinal manipulation: A comparative study.' *The Spine Journal* 3(3), 204–212. Available at www.ncbi.nlm.nih.gov/pubmed/14589201

Dishman, J.D., Ball, K.A. and Burke, J. (2002) 'First prize: Central motor excitability changes after spinal manipulation: A transcranial magnetic stimulation study.' *Journal of Manipulative and Physiological Therapeutics* 25(1), 1–9. Available at www.ncbi.nlm.nih.gov/pubmed/11898013

Dishman, J.D., Burke, J.R. and Dougherty, P. (2018) 'Motor neuron excitability attenuation as a sequel to lumbosacral manipulation in subacute low back pain patients and asymptomatic adults: A cross-sectional H-reflex study.' *Journal of Manipulative and Physiological Therapeutics* 41(5), 363–371. Available at www.ncbi.nlm.nih.gov/pubmed/29997032

Dishman, J.D., Cunningham, B.M. and Burke, J. (2002) 'Comparison of tibial nerve H-reflex excitability after cervical and lumbar spine manipulation.' *Journal of Manipulative and Physiological Therapeutics* 25(5), 318–325. Available at www.ncbi.nlm.nih.gov/pubmed/12072852

Dishman, J.D., Dougherty, P.E. and Burke, J.R. (2005) 'Evaluation of the effect of postural perturbation on motoneuronal activity following various methods of lumbar spinal manipulation.' *The Spine Journal* 5(6), 650–659. Available at www.ncbi.nlm.nih.gov/pubmed/16291107

Dishman, J.D., Greco, D.S. and Burke, J.R. (2008) 'Motor-evoked potentials recorded from lumbar erector spinae muscles: A study of corticospinal excitability changes associated with spinal manipulation.' *Journal of Manipulative and Physiological Therapeutics* 31(4), 258–270. Available at www.ncbi.nlm.nih.gov/pubmed/18486746

Downie, A.S., Vemulpad, S. and Bull, P.W. (2010) 'Quantifying the high-velocity, low-amplitude spinal manipulative thrust: A systematic review.' *Journal of Manipulative and Physiological Therapeutics* 33(7), 542–553. Available at www.ncbi.nlm.nih.gov/pubmed/20937432

Elenkov, I.J., Wilder, R.L., Chrousos, G.P. and Vizi, E.S. (2000) 'The sympathetic nerve – An integrative interface between two supersystems: The brain and the immune system.' *Pharmacological Reviews* 52(4), 595–638. Available at www.ncbi.nlm.nih.gov/pubmed/11121511

Evans, D.W. (2002) 'Mechanisms and effects of spinal high-velocity, low-amplitude thrust manipulation: Previous theories.' *Journal of Manipulative and Physiological Therapeutics* 25(4), 251–262. Available at www.ncbi.nlm.nih.gov/pubmed/12021744

Evans, D.W. and Breen, A.C. (2006) 'A biomechanical model for mechanically efficient cavitation production during spinal manipulation: Prethrust position and the neutral zone.' *Journal of Manipulative and Physiological Therapeutics* 29(1), 72–82. Available at www.ncbi.nlm.nih.gov/pubmed/16396734

Ferreira, M.L., Ferreira, P.H. and Hodges, P.W. (2007) 'Changes in postural activity of the trunk muscles following spinal manipulative therapy.' *Manual Therapy* 12(3), 240–248. Available at www.ncbi.nlm.nih.gov/pubmed/17452118

Frantzis, E., Druelle, P., Ross, K. and McGill, S. (2015) 'The accuracy of osteopathic manipulations of the lumbar spine: A pilot study.' *International Journal of Osteopathic Medicine* 18(1), 33–39. Available at www.sciencedirect.com/science/article/pii/S174606891400090X

Fryer, G. and Pearce, A.J. (2012) 'The effect of lumbosacral manipulation on corticospinal and spinal reflex excitability on asymptomatic participants.' *Journal of Manipulative and Physiological Therapeutics* 35(2), 86–93. Available at www.ncbi.nlm.nih.gov/pubmed/22036580

Funabashi, M., Kawchuk, G.N., Vette, A.H., Goldsmith, P. and Prasad, N. (2016) 'Tissue loading created during spinal manipulation in comparison to loading created by passive spinal movements.' *Scientific Reports* 6, 38107. Available at www.ncbi.nlm.nih.gov/pubmed/27905508

Geisser, M.E., Haig, A.J., Wallbom, A.S. and Wiggert, E.A. (2004) 'Pain-related fear, lumbar flexion, and dynamic EMG among persons with chronic musculoskeletal low back pain.' *The Clinical Journal of Pain* 20(2), 61–69. Available at www.ncbi.nlm.nih.gov/pubmed/14770044

George, S.Z., Bishop, M.D., Bialosky, J.E., Zeppieri, G. and Robinson, M.E. (2006) 'Immediate effects of spinal manipulation on thermal pain sensitivity: An experimental study.' *BMC Musculoskeletal Disorders* 7, 68. Available at www.ncbi.nlm.nih.gov/pubmed/16911795

Giles, P.D., Hensel, K.L., Pacchia, C.F. and Smith, M.L. (2013) 'Suboccipital decompression enhances heart rate variability indices of cardiac control in healthy subjects.' *The Journal of Alternative and Complementary Medicine* 19(2), 92–96. Available at www.ncbi.nlm.nih.gov/pubmed/22994907

Herrero, J.F., Laird, J.M. and Lopez-Garcia, J.A. (2000) 'Wind-up of spinal cord neurones and pain sensation: Much ado about something?' *Progress in Neurobiology* 61(2), 169–203. Available at www.ncbi.nlm.nih.gov/pubmed/10704997

Herzog, W. (2000) *Clinical Biomechanics of Spinal Manipulation.* London: Churchill Livingstone. Available at www.elsevier.com/books/clinical-biomechanics-of-spinal-manipulation/herzog/978-0-443-07808-8

Hodges, P.W. and Moseley, G.L. (2003) 'Pain and motor control of the lumbopelvic region: Effect and possible mechanisms.' *Journal of Electromyography and Kinesiology* 13(4), 361–370. Available at www.ncbi.nlm.nih.gov/pubmed/12832166

Johansson, H. and Sojka, P. (1991) 'Pathophysiological mechanisms involved in genesis and spread of muscular tension in occupational muscle pain and in chronic musculoskeletal pain syndromes: A hypothesis.' *Medical Hypotheses* 35(3), 196–203. Available at www.ncbi.nlm.nih.gov/pubmed/1943863

Keller, T.S., Colloca, C.J. and Gunzburg, R. (2003) 'Neuromechanical characterization of in vivo lumbar spinal manipulation. Part I. Vertebral motion.' *Journal of Manipulative and Physiological Therapeutics* 26(9), 567–578. Available at www.ncbi.nlm.nih.gov/pubmed/14673406

Kenney, M.J. and Ganta, C.K. (2011) 'Autonomic nervous system and immune system interactions.' *Comprehensive Physiology* 4(3), 1177–1200. Available at www.ncbi.nlm.nih.gov/pubmed/24944034

Klomjai, W., Katz, R. and Lackmy-Vallée, A. (2015) 'Basic principles of transcranial magnetic stimulation (TMS) and repetitive TMS (rTMS).' *Annals of Physical and Rehabilitation Medicine* 58(4), 208–213. Available at www.ncbi.nlm.nih.gov/pubmed/26319963

Korr, I.M. (1975) 'Proprioceptors and somatic dysfunction.' *The Journal of the American Osteopathic Association* 74(7), 638–650. Available at www.ncbi.nlm.nih.gov/pubmed/124754

Korr, I.M. (2012) *The Neurobiologic Mechanisms in Manipulative Therapy.* Boston, MA: Springer. Available at www.springer.com/gp/book/9781468489040

Korr, I.M., Wright, H.M. and Thomas, P.E. (1962) 'Effects of experimental myofascial insults on cutaneous patterns of sympathetic activity in man.' *Acta Neurovegetativa* 23, 329–355. Available at www.ncbi.nlm.nih.gov/pubmed/14458531

Lehman, G. (2012) 'Kinesiological research: The use of surface electromyography for assessing the effects of spinal manipulation.' *Journal of Electromyography and Kinesiology* 22(5), 692–696. Available at www.ncbi.nlm.nih.gov/pubmed/22425147

Lehman, G.J. and McGill, S.M. (2001) 'Spinal manipulation causes variable spine kinematic and trunk muscle electromyographic responses.' *Clinical Biomechanics* 16(4), 293–299. Available at www.ncbi.nlm.nih.gov/pubmed/11358616

Lelic, D., Niazi, I.K., Holt, K., Jochumsen, M., Dremstrup, K., Yielder, P. *et al.* (2016) 'Manipulation of dysfunctional spinal joints affects sensorimotor integration in the prefrontal cortex: A brain source localization study.' *Neural Plasticity* 2016, 3704964. Available at www.ncbi.nlm.nih.gov/pubmed/27047694

Lewis, S., Holmes, P., Woby, S., Hindle, J. and Fowler, N. (2012) 'The relationships between measures of stature recovery, muscle activity and psychological factors in patients with chronic low back pain.' *Manual Therapy* 17(1), 27–33. Available at www.ncbi.nlm.nih.gov/pubmed/21903445

Lund, J.P., Donga, R., Widmer, C.G. and Stohler, C.S. (1991) 'The pain-adaptation model: A discussion of the relationship between chronic musculoskeletal pain and motor activity.' *Canadian Journal of Physiology and Pharmacology* 69(5), 683–694. Available at www.ncbi.nlm.nih.gov/pubmed/1863921

Maigne, J.Y. and Vautravers, P. (2003) 'Mechanism of action of spinal manipulative therapy.' *Joint Bone Spine* 70(5), 336–341. Available at www.ncbi.nlm.nih.gov/pubmed/14563460

Melzack, R. and Wall, P.D. (1965) 'Pain mechanisms: a new theory.' *Science* 150(3699), 971–979. Available at www.ncbi.nlm.nih.gov/pubmed/5320816

Millan, M., Leboeuf-Yde, C., Budgell, B. and Amorim, M.A. (2012) 'The effect of spinal manipulative therapy on experimentally induced pain: A systematic literature review.' *Chiropractic & Manual Therapies* 20(1), 26. Available at www.ncbi.nlm.nih.gov/pubmed/22883534

Nougarou, F., Pagé, I., Loranger, M., Dugas, C. and Descarreaux, M. (2016) 'Neuromechanical response to spinal manipulation therapy: Effects of a constant rate of force application.' *BMC Complementary and Alternative Medicine* 16(1), 161. Available at www.ncbi.nlm.nih.gov/pubmed/27249939

Ogura, T., Tashiro, M., Masud, M., Watanuki, S., Shibuya, K., Yamaguchi, K. *et al.* (2011) 'Cerebral metabolic changes in men after chiropractic spinal manipulation for neck pain.' *Alternative Therapies in Health & Medicine* 17(6), 12–17. Available at www.ncbi.nlm.nih.gov/pubmed/22314714

O'Neill, S., Ødegaard-Olsen, Ø. and Søvde, B. (2015) 'The effect of spinal manipulation on deep experimental muscle pain in healthy volunteers.' *Chiropractic & Manual Therapies* 23, 25. Available at www.ncbi.nlm.nih.gov/pubmed/26347808

Padayachy, K., Vawda, G.H., Shaik, J. and McCarthy, P.W. (2010) 'The immediate effect of low back manipulation on serum cortisol levels in adult males with mechanical low back pain.' *Clinical Chiropractic* 13(4), 246–252. Available at www.sciencedirect.com/science/article/pii/S1479235410001756

Pickar, J.G. (2002) 'Neurophysiological effects of spinal manipulation.' *The Spine Journal* 2(5), 357–371. Available at www.ncbi.nlm.nih.gov/pubmed/14589467

Pickar, J.G. and Bolton, P.S. (2012) 'Spinal manipulative therapy and somatosensory activation.' *Journal of Electromyography and Kinesiology* 22(5), 785–794. Available at www.ncbi.nlm.nih.gov/pmc/articles/PMC3399029

Plaza-Manzano, G., Molina, F., Lomas-Vega, R., Martínez-Amat, A., Achalandabaso, A. and Hita-Contreras, F. (2014) 'Changes in biochemical markers of pain perception and stress response after spinal manipulation.' *Journal of Orthopaedic & Sports Physical Therapy* 44(4), 231–239. Available at www.ncbi.nlm.nih.gov/pubmed/24450367

Pongratz, G. and Straub, R.H. (2014) 'The sympathetic nervous response in inflammation.' *Arthritis Research & Therapy* 16(6), 504. Available at www.ncbi.nlm.nih.gov/pubmed/25789375

Potter, L., McCarthy, C.J. and Oldham, J.A. (2005) 'Physiological effects of spinal manipulation: A review of proposed theories.' *Physical Therapy Reviews* 10(3), 163–170. Available at www.researchgate.net/publication/233689100_Physiological_effects_of_spinal_manipulation_A_review_of_proposed_theories

Randoll, C., Gagnon-Normandin, V., Tessier, J., Bois, S., Rustamov, N., O'Shaughnessy, J. *et al.* (2017) 'The mechanism of back pain relief by spinal manipulation relies on decreased temporal summation of pain.' *Neuroscience* 349, 220–228. Available at www.ncbi.nlm.nih.gov/pubmed/28288900

Reed, W.R., Pickar, J.G., Sozio, R.S. and Long, C.R. (2014) 'Effect of spinal manipulation thrust magnitude on trunk mechanical activation thresholds of lateral thalamic neurons.' *Journal of Manipulative and Physiological Therapeutics* 37(5), 277–286. Available at www.ncbi.nlm.nih.gov/pubmed/24928636

Sampath, K.K., Mani, R., Cotter, J.D. and Tumilty, S. (2015) 'Measureable changes in the neuro-endocrinal mechanism following spinal manipulation.' *Medical Hypotheses* 85(6), 819–824. Available at www.ncbi.nlm.nih.gov/pubmed/26464145

Sampath, K.K., Botnmark, E., Mani, R., Cotter, J.D., Katare, R., Munasinghe, P.E. *et al.* (2017) 'Neuroendocrine response following a thoracic spinal manipulation in healthy men.' *Journal of Orthopaedic & Sports Physical Therapy* 47(9), 617–627. Available at www.ncbi.nlm.nih.gov/pubmed/28704625

Savva, C., Giakas, G. and Efstathiou, M. (2014) 'The role of the descending inhibitory pain mechanism in musculoskeletal pain following high-velocity, low amplitude thrust manipulation. A review of the literature.' *Journal of Back and Musculoskeletal Rehabilitation* 27(4), 377–382. Available at www.ncbi.nlm.nih.gov/pubmed/24867897

Schmid, A., Brunner, F., Wright, A. and Bachmann, L.M. (2008) 'Paradigm shift in manual therapy? Evidence for a central nervous system component in the response to passive cervical joint mobilisation.' *Manual Therapy* 13(5), 387–396. Available at www.ncbi.nlm.nih.gov/pubmed/18316238

Seffinger, M.A., Najm, W.I., Mishra, S.I., Adams, A., Dickerson, V.M., Murphy, L.S. *et al.* (2004) 'Reliability of spinal palpation for diagnosis of back and neck pain: A systematic review of the literature.' *Spine* 29(19), E413–E425. Available at www.ncbi.nlm.nih.gov/pubmed/15454722/

Sillevis, R., Cleland, J., Hellman, M. and Beekhuizen, K. (2010) 'Immediate effects of a thoracic spine thrust manipulation on the autonomic nervous system: A randomized clinical trial.' *Journal of Manual & Manipulative Therapy* 18(4), 181–190. Available at www.ncbi.nlm.nih.gov/pubmed/22131791

Skyba, D.A., Radhakrishnan, R., Rohlwing, J.J., Wright, A. and Sluka, K.A. (2003) 'Joint manipulation reduces hyperalgesia by activation of monoamine receptors but not opioid or GABA receptors in the spinal cord.' *Pain* 106(1–2), 159–168. Available at www.ncbi.nlm.nih.gov/pubmed/14581123

Song, X.J., Gan, Q., Cao, J.L., Wang, Z.B. and Rupert, R.L. (2006) 'Spinal manipulation reduces pain and hyperalgesia after lumbar intervertebral foramen inflammation in the rat.' *Journal of Manipulative and Physiological Therapeutics* 29(1), 5–13. Available at www.ncbi.nlm.nih.gov/pubmed/16396724

Sparks, C., Cleland, J.A., Elliott, J.M., Zagardo, M. and Liu, W.C. (2013) 'Using functional magnetic resonance imaging to determine if cerebral hemodynamic responses to pain change following thoracic spine thrust manipulation in healthy individuals.' *Journal of Orthopaedic & Sports Physical Therapy* 43(5), 340–348. Available at www.ncbi.nlm.nih.gov/pubmed/23485766

Staud, R., Craggs, J.G., Robinson, M.E., Perlstein, W.M. and Price, D.D. (2007) 'Brain activity related to temporal summation of C-fiber evoked pain.' *Pain* 129(1–2), 130–142. Available at www.ncbi.nlm.nih.gov/pubmed/17156923

Sterling, M., Jull, G. and Wright, A. (2001) 'Cervical mobilisation: Concurrent effects on pain, sympathetic nervous system activity and motor activity.' *Manual Therapy* 6(2), 72–81. Available at www.ncbi.nlm.nih.gov/pubmed/11414776

Suter, E., McMorland, G. and Herzog, W. (2005) 'Short-term effects of spinal manipulation on H-reflex amplitude in healthy and symptomatic subjects.' *Journal of Manipulative and Physiological Therapeutics* 28(9), 667–672. Available at www.ncbi.nlm.nih.gov/pubmed/16326236

Taylor, H.H. and Murphy, B. (2010) 'Altered central integration of dual somatosensory input after cervical spine manipulation.' *Journal of Manipulative and Physiological Therapeutics* 33(3), 178–188. Available at www.ncbi.nlm.nih.gov/pubmed/20350670

Travell, J., Rinzler, S. and Herman, M. (1942) 'Pain and disability of the shoulder and arm: Treatment by intramuscular infiltration with procaine hydrochloride.' *Journal of the American Medical Association* 120(6), 417–422. Available at https://jamanetwork.com/journals/jama/article-abstract/257842

Trompetto, C., Marinelli, L., Mori, L., Pelosin, E., Currà, A., Molfetta, L. *et al.* (2014) 'Pathophysiology of spasticity: Implications for neurorehabilitation.' *BioMed Research International* 2014, 354906. Available at www.ncbi.nlm.nih.gov/pubmed/25530960

Ulrich-Lai, Y.M. and Herman, J.P. 'Neural regulation of endocrine and autonomic stress responses.' *Nature Reviews Neuroscience* 10(6), 397–409. Available at www.ncbi.nlm.nih.gov/pubmed/19469025

van Dieën, J.H., Selen, L.P. and Cholewicki, J. (2003) 'Trunk muscle activation in low-back pain patients, an analysis of the literature.' *Journal of Electromyography and Kinesiology* 13(4), 333–351. Available at www.ncbi.nlm.nih.gov/pubmed/12832164

Vernon, H. (2000) 'Qualitative review of studies of manipulation-induced hypoalgesia.' *Journal of Manipulative and Physiological Therapeutics* 23(2), 134–138. Available at www.ncbi.nlm.nih.gov/pubmed/10714544

Walker, B.F., Koppenhaver, S.L., Stomski, N.J. and Hebert, J.J. (2015) 'Interrater reliability of motion palpation in the thoracic spine.' *Evidence-Based Complementary and Alternative Medicine* 2015, 815407. Available at www.ncbi.nlm.nih.gov/pubmed/26170883

Ward, J., Coats, J., Tyer, K., Weigand, S. and Williams, G. (2013) 'Immediate effects of anterior upper thoracic spine manipulation on cardiovascular response.' *Journal of Manipulative and Physiological Therapeutics* 36(2), 101–110. Available at www.ncbi.nlm.nih.gov/pubmed/23499145

Welch, A. and Boone, R. (2008) 'Sympathetic and parasympathetic responses to specific diversified adjustments to chiropractic vertebral subluxations of the cervical and thoracic spine.' *Journal of Chiropractic Medicine* 7(3), 86–93. Available at www.ncbi.nlm.nih.gov/pubmed/19646369

Wilder, D.G., Aleksiev, A.R., Magnusson, M.L., Pope, M.H., Spratt, K.F. and Goel, V.K. (1996) 'Muscular response to sudden load: A tool to evaluate fatigue and rehabilitation.' *Spine* 21(22), 2628–2639. Available at www.ncbi.nlm.nih.gov/pubmed/9045348

Williams, N.H., Hendry, M., Lewis, R., Russell, I., Westmoreland, A. and Wilkinson, C. (2007) 'Psychological response in spinal manipulation (PRISM): A systematic review of psychological outcomes in randomised controlled trials.' *Complementary Therapies in Medicine* 15(4), 271–283. Available at www.ncbi.nlm.nih.gov/pubmed/18054729

Win, N.N., Jorgensen, A.M., Chen, Y.S. and Haneline, M.T. (2015) 'Effects of upper and lower cervical spinal manipulative therapy on blood pressure and heart rate variability in volunteers and patients with neck pain: A randomized controlled, cross-over, preliminary study.' *Journal of Chiropractic Medicine* 14(1), 1–9. Available at www.ncbi.nlm.nih.gov/pubmed/26693212

Wright, A. (1995) 'Hypoalgesia post-manipulative therapy: A review of a potential neurophysiological mechanism.' *Manual Therapy* 1(1), 11–16. Available at www.ncbi.nlm.nih.gov/pubmed/11327789

Younes, M., Nowakowski, K., Didier-Laurent, B., Gombert, M. and Cottin, F. (2017) 'Effect of spinal manipulative treatment on cardiovascular autonomic control in patients with acute low back pain.' *Chiropractic & Manual Therapies* 25, 33. Available at www.ncbi.nlm.nih.gov/pubmed/29214015

Zafereo, J. and Deschenes, B.K. (2015) 'The role of spinal manipulation in modifying central sensitization.' *Journal of Applied Biobehavioral Research* 20(2), 84–99. Available at www.researchgate.net/publication/277560942_The_Role_of_Spinal_Manipulation_in_Modifying_Central_Sensitization

Zedka, M., Prochazka, A., Knight, B., Gillard, D. and Gauthier, M. (1999) 'Voluntary and reflex control of human back muscles during induced pain.' *The Journal of Physiology* 520(2), 591–604. Available at www.ncbi.nlm.nih.gov/pubmed/10523425

Zegarra-Parodi, R., Park, P.Y., Heath, D.M., Makin, I.R., Degenhardt, B.F. and Roustit, M. (2015) 'Assessment of skin blood flow following spinal manual therapy: A systematic review.' *Manual Therapy* 20(2), 228–249. Available at www.ncbi.nlm.nih.gov/pubmed/25261088

Zhang, J., Dean, D., Nosco, D., Strathopulos, D. and Floros, M. (2006) 'Effect of chiropractic care on heart rate variability and pain in a multisite clinical study.' *Journal of Manipulative and Physiological Therapeutics* 29(4), 267–274. Available at www.ncbi.nlm.nih.gov/pubmed/16690380

2

CAN MANIPULATION AFFECT THE VISCERAL ORGANS?

Introduction

Spinal manipulation is a non-invasive treatment option for the management of musculoskeletal pain and disability. It has been proven to be a safe and effective therapy if applied skilfully and appropriately. To date, however, little scientific evidence exists in support of its use in non-musculoskeletal complaints. While proponents of spinal manipulation claim the therapy to be similarly effective for visceral disorders, critics have labelled the claim controversial due to a lack of robust neurobiological rationale. This chapter therefore looks at the proposed theories concerning visceral responses of spinal manipulation, and reviews the associated physiological evidence.

Current theoretical basis

Spinal manipulation, by definition, is a specific form of manual therapy; hence, it theoretically adheres to the same philosophy and principles of spinal manipulative therapy. Unlike physicians of the conventional medical system, therapists of spinal manipulation treat their patients with a holistic approach – as a unit of body, mind and soul. They consider the body as a whole integrated organism in which all parts function interdependently, and prioritise spinal integrity as an indicator for the wellbeing of an individual. Hence, manual therapists believe that the good health of a person depends on the smooth functioning of all structures in the body, including bones, muscles, tendons, ligaments and organs. By manipulating a patient's muscles or joints, therapists tend to aid the body's self-healing ability, correcting the structural anomalies (Di Fabio 1992; Vickers and Zollman 1999).

Several studies have confirmed that manipulation of the spine can influence some organ functions (Bakris *et al.* 2007; Budgell 1999; Hawk *et al.* 2007). However, it is not yet known how spinal manipulation affects visceral function, and whether these effects are clinically relevant in the treatment of visceral diseases. Most of the early theories concerning the effect of manipulation on the visceral system are largely focused on vitalism. Recent theories propose that all organs and structures of the body slide and glide with an interconnected synchronicity, as the whole body is enveloped by an uninterrupted network of connective tissue known as fascia (Hall 2012). Accordingly, the visceral system depends on this synchronicity to function smoothly. In healthy individuals, this harmony remains stable regardless of our body's endless variations in motion. But when the synchronicity in movement is affected due to formation of adhesions or abnormal muscle tone, it results in an erratic tension between organs, and ultimately limits the body's normal range of motion. This, in turn, leads to disease and dysfunction of various systems of the body.

Therapists of spinal manipulation claim to correct this disharmony by first locating the source of the problem through palpation, and then realigning changes in the biomechanical dynamics (e.g., position and movement faults) by manipulation. However, many critics of spinal manipulation have rejected such a claim, since there is no direct neural connection between the spine and visceral system. Some have even remarked that the claim is completely unrealistic, arguing that visceral tissues do not depend on spinal nerve root signals to run themselves. In addition, organs could function smoothly on their own, even if a spinal nerve root is cut. Hence, the critics mainly argue that there is no justifiable reason that spinal manipulation can address visceral disorders. In support of this argument, they also say that spinal manipulation has a valid concept in treating musculoskeletal disorders, as musculoskeletal structures rely on the nerves that pass between vertebrae (Ingraham 2017).

No neurological connection between the spine and organs: A brief rebuttal

It is undeniable what the critics of spinal manipulation argue concerning its neurophysiological limitations in addressing visceral disorders. But we strongly disagree with the argument that manipulation has no reasonable theoretical basis to modulate visceral function. Although the corpus of literature is small, there is some evidence that spinal manipulation is beneficial for certain visceral disorders (Bakris *et al.* 2007; Budgell 1999). We agree that a comprehensive neurobiological rationale is still missing to justify our claim. However, this is not due to there being no neurological connection between the visceral system and the spine, but because of the limited interests of case studies and controlled trials in exploring neural mechanisms (Bolton and Budgell 2012). So far, only a few basic physiological studies in humans have been done to determine the mechanisms underlying the visceral responses of spinal manipulation. Some authors have already attributed these responses to somato-autonomic reflexes (Jowsey and Perry 2010; Moulson and Watson 2006; Perry *et al.* 2011). While this is not unreasonable, others have suggested alternative mechanisms such as an involvement of somato-humoral pathways (Bolton and Budgell 2012).

The autonomic nervous system (ANS) controls the involuntary bodily responses. It regulates and supplies various organs of the viscera such as the heart, kidneys, liver, lungs and digestive glands. The ANS also has potential interaction with the nociceptive (pain) system on multiple levels, which include the brain stem, fore brain, periphery and dorsal horn (Benarroch 2006). Therefore, any intervention that influences the functions of the ANS has significant clinical relevance. The effects of spinal manipulation on the ANS are well established in the literature. This has been demonstrated using various outcome measures such as heart rate variability, pupillary reflex and skin blood flow indexes (Bolton and Budgell 2012; Sampath et al. 2015). In addition, several studies done to investigate the neuroendocrine responses have reported a manipulation-induced increase in serum cortisol levels (Padayachy et al. 2010; Plaza-Manzano et al. 2014). Hence, in the theorised mechanisms of spinal manipulation, the peripheral sympathetic nervous system (PSNS) has been given a prominent role in the modulation of pain and inflammation.

Furthermore, after reviewing a range of mechanistic studies, Sampath et al. (2015) hypothesised that spinal manipulation might co-activate both the ANS and endocrine system. Since these two systems have been reported to work together, the authors suggested that post-manipulation changes in the ANS might be accompanied by changes in the function of the hypothalamic–pituitary–adrenal (HPA) axis. They also proposed a possible neural framework in support of their hypothesis. Taken together, it can be said that the autonomically mediated responses and the somato-humoural pathways are justifiable areas of research to demonstrate the visceral effects of spinal manipulation. In addition, it is totally baseless to say that mechanical stimulation of the spine has no neurobiological basis to influence the visceral organs. Even if there is no direct neural connection between the body's organs and the spine, spinal manipulation could indirectly result in measurable changes in the visceral system mediated by the ANS.

Misunderstanding, or intentional misinterpretation?

Some critics are so critical about spinal manipulation, as if nothing 'good' can be expected from it! They find unthinkable problems in the basic philosophy and principles of manipulation, and consider every theoretical explanation to be flawed, no matter the evidence against them. One common argument of these critics against the use of spinal manipulation in visceral disorders is that organs are not affected even if a spinal nerve root is completely cut, so there is no valid point in using the therapy. Is this really so?

It is true that the complete loss of a spinal nerve root will certainly paralyse something in the musculoskeletal structure, but not a visceral organ. However, this does not mean organs are not affected at all, even if a serious spinal injury occurs. After a major spinal nerve injury, organs will continue to run smoothly for a short duration, but the long-term fate of them is scary. There will, in fact, be autonomic dysregulation over time, which will gradually lead to organ dysfunction and make matters worse for overall systemic health (Sezer, Akkuş and Uğurlu 2015; Stein *et al.* 2010). This actually proves the oldest philosophy of spinal manipulation, that all organs and structures in the body work interdependently, and that spinal health is critical for their smooth functioning. Moreover, because spinal manipulation has been reported to influence various functions of the ANS, the argument that manipulation cannot affect visceral function becomes invalid, although these effects are indirect.

On the other hand, we believe the critics have also misunderstood the very concept on which therapists of spinal manipulation treat visceral disorders. The basic theory of visceral manipulation, that all the body's organs and structures move with an interconnected synchronicity, is actually based on fascia, not on nerve supply from the spine to the organs. A fascia is an interconnected network of fibrous collagenous tissues that has the ability to adjust its elasticity and consistency under tension (Findley *et al.* 2012). It supports the body in a number of ways, by:

- providing ongoing physiological support for the body's metabolically active systems composed of specialised cells and tissues

- connecting, communicating and coordinating all parts of the body in its entirety

- contributing to haemodynamic and biochemical processes

- assisting in response to mechanical stress

- maintaining posture and locomotion

- facilitating movements.

The effects of spinal manipulation on fascia have been confirmed in the current literature. Manipulation has been reported to breach fascial crosslinks, ease fascial tightness and normalise fascial motion (Harper, Steinbeck and Aron 2016; Oulianova 2011; Simmonds, Miller and Gemmell 2012). Therefore, we conclude that it is unreasonable to find problems with our claim that manipulation corrects disharmony in visceral movement.

In conclusion, we suggest that before labelling a claim controversial, the critics need first to thoroughly understand the therapeutic goals behind the mechanical stimulation of the spine. Unlike a conventional intervention, spinal manipulation is not a curative therapy. The ultimate goal of this therapy is to create the best possible environment for the body's own self-healing mechanisms. Hence, by affecting visceral function via the ANS and releasing fascial restrictions, therapists of spinal manipulation are actually sending 'SOS' signals to the brain and paving the way so that the body can self-heal on its own.

References

Bakris, G., Dickholtz Sr, M., Meyer, P.M., Kravitz, G., Avery, E., Miller, M. *et al.* (2007) 'Atlas vertebra realignment and achievement of arterial pressure goal in hypertensive patients: A pilot study.' *Journal of Human Hypertension 21*(5), 347.

Benarroch, E.E. (2006) 'Pain-autonomic interactions.' *Neurological Sciences 27*(Suppl. 2), S130–S133. Available at www.ncbi.nlm.nih.gov/pubmed/16688616

Bolton, P.S. and Budgell, B. (2012) 'Visceral responses to spinal manipulation.' *Journal of Electromyography and Kinesiology 22*(5), 777–784.

Budgell, B.S. (1999) 'Spinal manipulative therapy and visceral disorders.' *Chiropractic Journal of Australia 29*, 123–128.

Di Fabio, R.P. (1992) 'Efficacy of manual therapy.' *Physical Therapy 72*(12), 853–864.

Findley, T., Chaudhry, H., Stecco, A. and Roman, M. (2012) 'Fascia research – A narrative review.' *Journal of Bodywork and Movement Therapies 16*(1), 67–75.

Hall, H. (2012) 'Visceral Manipulation Embraced by the APTA.' Science-Based Medicine. Available at https://sciencebasedmedicine.org/visceral-manipulation-embraced-by-the-apta

Harper, B., Steinbeck, L. and Aron, A. (2016) 'The effect of adding Fascial Manipulation® to the physical therapy plan of care for low back pain patients.' *Journal of Bodywork and Movement Therapies 1*(20), 148–149.

Hawk, C., Khorsan, R., Lisi, A.J., Ferrance, R.J. and Evans, M.W. (2007) 'Chiropractic care for nonmusculoskeletal conditions: A systematic review with implications for whole systems research.' *The Journal of Alternative and Complementary Medicine 13*(5), 491–512.

Ingraham, P. (2017) 'Spinal nerve roots do not hook up to organs!' PainScience.com. Available at www.painscience.com/articles/spinal-nerves-and-organs.php

Jowsey, P. and Perry, J. (2010) 'Sympathetic nervous system effects in the hands following a grade III postero-anterior rotatory mobilisation technique applied to T4: A randomised, placebo-controlled trial.' *Manual Therapy 15*(3), 248–253.

Moulson, A. and Watson, T. (2006) 'A preliminary investigation into the relationship between cervical snags and sympathetic nervous system activity in the upper limbs of an asymptomatic population.' *Manual Therapy 11*(3), 214–224.

Oulianova, I. (2011) 'An Investigation into the Effects of Fascial Manipulation on Dysmenorrhea.' Doctoral dissertation, RMTBC.

Padayachy, K., Vawda, G.H.M., Shaik, J. and McCarthy, P.W. (2010) 'The immediate effect of low back manipulation on serum cortisol levels in adult males with mechanical low back pain.' *Clinical Chiropractic 13*(4), 246–252.

Perry, J., Green, A., Singh, S. and Watson, P. (2011) 'A preliminary investigation into the magnitude of effect of lumbar extension exercises and a segmental rotatory manipulation on sympathetic nervous system activity.' *Manual Therapy* 16(2), 190–195.

Plaza-Manzano, G., Molina, F., Lomas-Vega, R., Martínez-Amat, A., Achalandabaso, A. and Hita-Contreras, F. (2014) 'Changes in biochemical markers of pain perception and stress response after spinal manipulation.' *Journal of Orthopaedic & Sports Physical Therapy* 44(4), 231–239.

Sampath, K.K., Mani, R., Cotter, J.D. and Tumilty, S. (2015) 'Measureable changes in the neuro-endocrinal mechanism following spinal manipulation.' *Medical Hypotheses* 85(6), 819–824.

Sezer, N., Akkuş, S. and Uğurlu, F.G. (2015) 'Chronic complications of spinal cord injury.' *World Journal of Orthopedics* 6(1), 24.

Simmonds, N., Miller, P. and Gemmell, H. (2012) 'A theoretical framework for the role of fascia in manual therapy.' *Journal of Bodywork and Movement Therapies* 16(1), 83–93.

Stein, D.M., Menaker, J., McQuillan, K., Handley, C., Aarabi, B. and Scalea, T.M. (2010) 'Risk factors for organ dysfunction and failure in patients with acute traumatic cervical spinal cord injury.' *Neurocritical Care* 13(1), 29–39.

Vickers, A. and Zollman, C. (1999) 'ABC of complementary medicine: The manipulative therapies: Osteopathy and chiropractic.' *British Medical Journal* 319(7218), 1176.

3

MOTION PALPATION MISCONCEPTIONS

Introduction

Spinal motion palpation is an integral diagnostic procedure that has been widely used by manual therapy practitioners to diagnose spinal dysfunction. It is frequently used to locate primary areas of joint restriction, asymmetries in spinal level and intersegmental hypomobility and hypermobility. It helps determine whether a patient needs spinal manipulation, and, if so, where to apply the thrust (Bergmann and Peterson 2010). Motion palpation is also performed to detect functional changes in other regions (e.g., shoulder or hip) related to the spine. In addition, a recent study among physiotherapists in Australia reported that around 98 per cent of the respondents were using manual palpatory tests to take treatment decisions (Abbott *et al.* 2009).

Over the last century, various palpatory techniques have been developed to detect different degrees of motion restriction at the spinal level. However, the clinical utility of these palpation techniques in the assessment of spinal dysfunction has been controversial (Walker *et al.* 2015). Although proponents of manual therapy consider it to be a valid and reliable indicator of spinal abnormalities, a majority of studies have found it to be unreliable due to low indices of agreement (Cooperstein and Young 2016; Haneline *et al.* 2008; Huijbregts 2002; Walker *et al.* 2015). Because the reliability of an examination tool is a prerequisite for its clinical utility, the use of motion palpation to guide treatment interventions is questionable.

This chapter is therefore written to improve our understanding concerning the validity and reliability of spinal motion palpation.

Intrarater and interrater reliability of motion palpation

In the context of spinal motion palpation, reliability refers to the degree of consistency in the diagnostic outcomes when it is repeated under identical conditions. Intrarater reliability is the degree of agreement obtained by the same rater across two or more trials using the same procedure. Interrater reliability is the relative consistency of agreement among two or more raters concerning the outcomes of the same procedure (Watkins and Portney 2009).

Over the past decades, a large body of research has been conducted to determine the reliability of motion palpation. However, the reliability estimates have been reported to vary widely from study to study (Walker *et al.* 2015). The literature investigating the intrarater reliability using κ values suggested the degree of agreement to be moderate. On the other hand, the interrater reliability of motion palpation has been found to be poor, often the agreement at near chance levels (Haneline *et al.* 2008). Huijbregts (2002) proposed that this higher intra- than interrater reliability might be due to incorrect detection of the vertebral level by the raters at which motion restriction was identified. Nyberg and Russell Smith (2013) stated that a therapist's primary focus during motion palpation might also be responsible for the low level of agreement between raters. They suggested that some therapists might solely concentrate on the degree of spinal displacement while others might be more focused on assessing the velocity of the displacement.

Systematic reviews done to assess the quality of motion palpation studies have found significant statistical and methodological shortcomings in the majority of these studies (Stochkendahl *et al.* 2006; van Trijffel *et al.* 2005). In a recent systematic review by Haneline *et al.* (2008), it was found that only 4 out of 44 retrieved articles were of acceptable quality. Some of the common methodological flaws in these studies included poor patient selection, inexperienced raters, use of irrelevant rating scales and low levels of reproducibility. Moreover, in most of the earlier studies, therapists were not allowed to detect different degrees of spinal stiffness, which obviously affected the level of agreement between them (Cooperstein and Young 2016). However, despite these limitations, the majority of high-quality studies have reported poor interrater reliability of motion palpation. The level of interrater agreement is usually found to be no better than chance.

Here are some of the most likely reasons for the low reliability of motion palpation:

- differences in palpatory testing procedures

- inaccurate interpretation of motion abnormality at the segmental level

- incorrect identification of spinal landmarks

- anatomical difference between patients.

Alternatively, Cooperstein and Young (2016) opined that significant interrater agreement could be achieved with motion palpation if continuous analysis is performed and the findings are stratified by therapist confidence. They suggested that instead of performing the segmental level-by-level evaluation to identify spinal stiffness, therapists should focus on finding the stiffest site and use their confidence as a surrogate measure to determine the degree of spinal stiffness.

Bracht *et al.* (2015) also suggested that the therapist's lack of confidence with the test result might be a variable affecting the interrater agreement.

Reliability of osteopathic motion palpation tests

The osteopathic approach of motion palpation adheres to the principles of Fryette's Laws, which is a set of three laws that serve as guiding principles for osteopaths to differentiate between spinal dysfunctions. These laws suggest that the existence of a somatic dysfunction in one plane of the spine will negatively affect vertebral motion in all other planes (DiGiovanna, Schiowitz and Dowling 2005). The first two laws assume that when one or more vertebrae are out of alignment, the vertebral movement will be toward the side that has more freedom of movement. For example, according to the first law, if there is an asymmetry in the position of T3 and T4 vertebrae, side bending to the right will cause a simultaneous horizontal rotation to the left. In brief, these laws imply that the vertebra has a natural tendency to position itself opposite to the side with less mobility (Nelson and Glonek 2007).

Studies done to understand the mechanical dysfunctions of vertebrae have reported a decrease in spinal joint movement in patients with low back pain (LBP). Passias *et al.* (2011), whose aim was to quantify abnormal vertebral motion, found greater segmental hypermobility and hypomobility in discogenic LBP patients compared with asymptomatic normal subjects. Furthermore, although Snider *et al.* (2008) did not find a significant difference between chronic LBP and non-LBP groups for the incidence of static rotational asymmetry, they reported a greater asymmetry in chronic LBP patients than those without LBP. These findings further highlight the significance of identifying rotational asymmetry and the potential of some palpatory tests that can detect asymmetrical vertebral position.

Osteopaths frequently use a motion palpation test to identify the rotational asymmetry of the vertebrae in the transverse plane. The vertebral rotation test is usually performed to detect whether there is asymmetry in the vertebral position and to determine the severity of somatic dysfunction. So far, only a few studies have investigated the intra- and interrater reliability of palpatory tests that assess rotational vertebral asymmetries (Degenhardt *et al.* 2005, 2010; Holmgren and Waling 2008). However, the findings of these studies are contradictory and do not suggest motion palpation as a reliable test to identify vertebral asymmetry. Recently, to confirm the results of earlier studies, Bracht *et al.* (2015) assessed the rotational movement asymmetry of the lumbar vertebrae using a motion palpation test in order to determine its intra- and interrater reliability. Similar to previous authors, they also found low inter- and intrarater agreement of the motion palpation test used. Taken together, it can be said that the reliability of palpatory tests for the assessment of vertebral rotational asymmetry is questionable.

Conclusion and recommendations

Motion palpation tests have a wide clinical use in manual therapy. However, since the reliability of these tests has been questionable, clinicians should follow the current clinical recommendations for the assessment of spinal dysfunction. Based on the conclusions made by the studies reviewed, we developed the following suggestions for therapists:

- *Have a qualitative approach.* When assessing a patient, the therapist should focus more on the quality of motion with end-range spinal motions than the quantity of movement in the palpated segments. This is because it is clinically more important to detect the presence of a motion abnormality than the exact segmental level at which the abnormality was found. The therapist's decision to provide a spinal manipulation largely depends on whether there is a motion restriction at the spinal level and the symptoms reproduced with the palpation test. Huijbregts (2002) suggested that incorrect identification of the segmental level with abnormality might be a possible explanation for the low interrater agreement. Moreover, the systematic review by Haneline *et al.* (2008) found that studies that reported fair agreement favoured the qualitative or passive palpation method more than the quantitative approach.

- *Consider using pain provocation tests.* In addition to using a more passive motion palpation test, the therapist should focus on pain response with provocation of the involved spinal segments. Pain provocation tests have been shown to demonstrate higher levels of reliability than motion palpation for identifying spinal dysfunction and instability (Hicks *et al.* 2003; Malanga, Landes and Nadler 2003; Telli, Telli and Topal 2018). On the other hand, Nyberg and Russell Smith (2013) suggested that the use of a passive palpation technique would help improve the therapist's tactile perception and ability to discriminate spinal motion behaviour.

References

Abbott, J.H., Flynn, T.W., Fritz, J.M., Hing, W.A., Reid, D. and Whitman, J.M. (2009) 'Manual physical assessment of spinal segmental motion: Intent and validity.' *Manual Therapy* 14(1), 36–44.

Bergmann, T.F. and Peterson, D.H. (2010) *Chiropractic Technique: Principles and Procedures.* St Louis, MO: Elsevier Health Sciences.

Bracht, M.A., Nunes, G.S., Celestino, J., Schwertner, D.S., França, L.C. and de Noronha, M. (2015) 'Inter- and intra-observer agreement of the motion palpation test for lumbar vertebral rotational asymmetry.' *Physiotherapy Canada* 67(2), 169–173.

Cooperstein, R. and Young, M. (2016) 'The reliability of spinal motion palpation determination of the location of the stiffest spinal site is influenced by confidence ratings: A secondary analysis of three studies.' *Chiropractic and Manual Therapies* 24(1), 50.

Degenhardt, B.F., Johnson, J.C., Snider, K.T. and Snider, E.J. (2010) 'Maintenance and improvement of interobserver reliability of osteopathic palpatory tests over a 4-month period.' *The Journal of the American Osteopathic Association* 110(10), 579–586.

Degenhardt, B.F., Snider, K.T., Snider, E.J. and Johnson, J.C. (2005) 'Interobserver reliability of osteopathic palpatory diagnostic tests of the lumbar spine: Improvements from consensus training.' *The Journal of the American Osteopathic Association* 105(10), 465–473.

DiGiovanna, E.L., Schiowitz, S. and Dowling, D.J. (eds) (2005) *An Osteopathic Approach to Diagnosis and Treatment.* Philadelphia, PA: Lippincott Williams & Wilkins.

Haneline, M.T., Cooperstein, R., Young, M. and Birkeland, K. (2008) 'Spinal motion palpation: A comparison of studies that assessed intersegmental end feel vs excursion.' *Journal of Manipulative and Physiological Therapeutics* 31(8), 616–626.

Hicks, G.E., Fritz, J.M., Delitto, A. and Mishock, J. (2003) 'Interrater reliability of clinical examination measures for identification of lumbar segmental instability.' *Archives of Physical Medicine and Rehabilitation* 84(12), 1858–1864.

Holmgren, U. and Waling, K. (2008) 'Inter-examiner reliability of four static palpation tests used for assessing pelvic dysfunction.' *Manual Therapy* 13(1), 50–56.

Huijbregts, P.A. (2002) 'Spinal motion palpation: A review of reliability studies.' *Journal of Manual and Manipulative Therapy* 10(1), 24–39.

Malanga, G.A., Landes, P. and Nadler, S.F. (2003) 'Provocative tests in cervical spine examination: Historical basis and scientific analyses.' *Pain Physician* 6(2), 199–206.

Nelson, K.E. and Glonek, T. (eds) (2007) *Somatic Dysfunction in Osteopathic Family Medicine.* Philadelphia, PA: Lippincott Williams & Wilkins.

Nyberg, R.E. and Russell Smith, A. (2013) 'The science of spinal motion palpation: A review and update with implications for assessment and intervention.' *Journal of Manual and Manipulative Therapy* 21(3), 160–167.

Passias, P.G., Wang, S., Kozanek, M., Xia, Q., Li, W., Grottkau, B. *et al.* (2011) 'Segmental lumbar rotation in patients with discogenic low back pain during functional weight-bearing activities.' *The Journal of Bone and Joint Surgery* 93(1), 29.

Snider, K.T., Johnson, J.C., Snider, E.J. and Degenhardt, B.F. (2008) 'Increased incidence and severity of somatic dysfunction in subjects with chronic low back pain.' *The Journal of the American Osteopathic Association* 108(8), 372–378.

Stochkendahl, M.J., Christensen, H.W., Hartvigsen, J., Vach, W., Haas, M., Hestbaek, L. *et al.* (2006) 'Manual examination of the spine: A systematic critical literature review of reproducibility.' *Journal of Manipulative and Physiological Therapeutics* 29(6), 475–485.

Telli, H., Telli, S. and Topal, M. (2018) 'The validity and reliability of provocation tests in the diagnosis of sacroiliac joint dysfunction.' *Pain Physician* 21(4), E367–E376.

van Trijffel, E., Anderegg, Q., Bossuyt, P.M.M. and Lucas, C. (2005) 'Inter-examiner reliability of passive assessment of intervertebral motion in the cervical and lumbar spine: A systematic review.' *Manual Therapy* 10(4), 256–269.

Walker, B.F., Koppenhaver, S.L., Stomski, N.J. and Hebert, J.J. (2015) 'Interrater reliability of motion palpation in the thoracic spine.' *Evidence-Based Complementary and Alternative Medicine* 2015, 815407. Available at www.ncbi.nlm.nih.gov/pubmed/26170883

Watkins, M.P. and Portney, L. (2009) *Foundations of Clinical Research: Applications to Practice.* Upper Saddle River, NJ: Pearson/Prentice Hall.

4

THE CERVICAL SPINE

Introduction

The cervical spine consists of the superior seven vertebrae of the vertebral column located between the occiput (O) and the first vertebra of the thoracic spine (T1). It is by far the most filigree part of the human spine and it serves the unique function of leveraging the head in space (König and Spetzger 2016; Souza 2016). The positioning of the head relative to the cervical spine may give occasion for injuries that may be treated by cervical spine manipulation (CSM). The CSM technique 'is a manual treatment where a vertebral joint is passively moved between the normal range of motion and the limits of its normal integrity' (Ernst 2007, pp.330–338). The technique is most frequently employed by chiropractors and to a lesser extent by other manual therapists and physicians (Ernst 2007).

Therapists use CSM to reduce pain and re-establish optimal function of the neck, but the treatment techniques employed have been associated with increased risk of severe adverse events (Yamamoto *et al.* 2018). A review of cases published over a five-year period suggested causal links between CSM and various vascular accidents and other non-vascular complications, often with serious consequences (Ernst 2007). A recent study comparing CSM and home exercise with advice and medication for the treatment of acute and subacute neck pain found no statistically relevant differences between the two manual treatment methods, further concluding that both had significantly more benefits in the short and long term over medication (Bronfort *et al.* 2012).

While there is an overall paucity of research on the effectiveness of CSM, growing safety concerns have driven the establishment of guiding principles for the teaching and practice of CSM (Yamamoto *et al.* 2018). An example of such a guideline is the 'International framework for examination of the cervical region for potential of cervical arterial dysfunction prior to orthopaedic manual therapy intervention' that was established to aid the therapist's clinical reasoning without being prescriptive (Rushton *et al.* 2014). It is imperative for therapists using CSM to familiarise themselves with these guidelines to minimise adverse outcomes following treatment.

This chapter explores the joints of the cervical spine and their range of motion, and it summarises special tests that may be employed in diagnosing serious pathology in the neck region. Common injuries to the cervical spine and red flags for CSM are discussed.

Joints

Anatomists often divide the cervical spine into two physiologically distinct regions identified as the upper cervical spine (O–C2) and the lower cervical spine (C3–C7) (Souza 2016). The upper segment allows for a greater degree of rotation owing to the unique morphology and articulation of the atlas and the axis (C1 and C2) (König and Spetzger 2016; Shen, Samartzis and Fessler 2015; Souza 2016). The atlas has an inimitable ring-like appearance due to the absence of a body, having an anterior tubercle instead. The axis, on the other hand, has an odontoid process referred to as the dens that projects superiorly to form a synovial joint with the posterior aspect of the atlas (Shen *et al.* 2015). The vertebrae of the lower segment (C3–C6) are very similar, consisting of a relatively broad body, transverse processes, pedicles and bifid, caudally projecting spinous processes (Shen *et al.* 2015; Standring 2016). Synovial intervertebral joints (facet joints) form between the superior articular process of one vertebra and the inferior articular process of the adjacent cranial vertebra, serving to guide and limit segmental motion (König and Spetzger 2016). The various joints are summarised in Table 4.1.

Table 4.1. Joints of the cervical spine

Joint name	Description	Function
Atlanto-occipital joint (O–C1)	• A synovial joint of ellipsoid variety • Forms due to articulation between the atlas and the occipital condyles • Made up of a pair of condyloid joints	• Responsible for 50% of total neck flexion and extension • Serves to maintain and support the weight and movement of the head and neck
Atlantoaxial joint (C1–C2)	• A complex joint that consists of three synovial joints • Forms due to articulation between the atlas and axis • Made up of a pair of plain joints (lateral joints) and a pivot joint (median joint)	• Responsible for 50% of all cervical rotation • Serves to maintain and support the weight and movement of the head and neck
Lower cervical joints (C3–C7)	• Originates from the inferior surface of the axis and ends at the superior surface of the first thoracic vertebra (T1) • Articulations include the uncovertebral joints, disc-vertebral body and facet joints	• Responsible for 50% of total neck flexion, extension and rotation

Sources: Johnson (1991); Standring (2016); White and Panjabi (1990)

Range of motion

The cervical spine enables a high degree of movement in six different directions: namely, anterior flexion, posterior extension, lateral bending to the left and right as well as rotation to the left and right (König and Spetzger 2016) (see Table 4.2). The various motions of the cervical spine under functional conditions are usually complex multi-dimensional combinations of these basic movements (König and Spetzger 2016). 'The cervical spine can rotate about 90°, laterally bend at 45°, forward flex to 60° and extend backward 75°' (Budd *et al.* 2017, p.155).

Table 4.2. Range of motion between different cervical joints

Motion unit	Range of motion
O–C1	• 25° of flexion and extension • 5° of axial rotation • 7° of lateral bending
C1–C2	• 15° of flexion and extension • 30° of axial rotation • 4° or less of lateral bending
C2–C3	• 8° of flexion and extension • 9° of rotation • 10° of lateral bending
C3–C4	• 13° of flexion and extension • 12° of rotation • 10° of lateral bending
C4–C5	• 19° of flexion and extension • 12° of rotation • 10° of lateral bending
C5–C6	• 17° of flexion and extension • 14° of rotation • 8° of lateral bending
C6–C7	• 16° of flexion and extension • 10° of rotation • 7° of lateral bending

Sources: Schafer and Faye (1990); Tubbs et al. *(2010, 2011)*

Common neck injuries

The positioning of the head balanced on the cervical spine creates a potentially injurious lever effect when the head is forced to move rapidly into extremes of flexion, extension or lateral flexion, as often happens in motor vehicle accidents and falls (Budd *et al.* 2017; Souza 2016). 'Some focal problems include cervical strain, sprain, internal disc disruption (discogenic pain), or cervical spinal degenerative change, cervical "whip-lash" syndrome, and myofascial pain' (Budd *et al.* 2017, p.156).

The sudden neck movements characteristic of CSM have been linked to spontaneous cervical artery dissection involving the vertebral arteries due to their proximity to the cervical spine (Kennell *et al.* 2017). Some recent case control studies have nevertheless found a similar association between chiropractic care and strokes when compared with treatment given by primary care physicians for headache and neck pain, suggesting that pre-existing pathologies may have a confounding effect on the outcome of CSM (Cassidy *et al.* 2008; Hutting *et al.* 2018; Kennell *et al.* 2017). See Table 4.3 below.

Table 4.3. Common injuries of the cervical joints

Common injuries	Characteristics
Atlanto-occipital dislocation	• This is a very unstable cranio-cervical injury associated with substantial neurological mortality and morbidity • Often linked with damage to the bony structures and ligaments linking the skull to the cervical spine • The dislocation may result from extreme extension or flexion, as is the case with motor vehicle accidents • Incidence of 8–31% in fatal traffic accidents and 10% in fatal cervical spine injuries
Jefferson fracture	• A fracture of the atlas (C1) produced by compressive downward force • One or both of the anterior or posterior arches are involved • Severe cases may involve the four aspects of the atlas ring • This accounts for approximately 25% of cranio-cervical injuries, 2–13% of injuries involving the cervical spine and 1.3% of spinal fractures

Common injuries	Characteristics
Odontoid fracture	• Most commonly occurs as a result of hyperextension of the cervical spine • May also result from hyperflexion of the cervical spine • Occurs at the base of the dens of C2 • Has a high non-union rate • Supplanting of the fractured segment may occur either anteriorly, posteriorly or laterally • Accounts for 10–15% of cervical spine fractures
Atlantoaxial instability	• A disorder of the atlantoaxial complex (C1 and C2) that limits neck rotation • Usually congenital, but may result from pathological relaxing of the transverse and adjacent ligaments or of the lateral atlantoaxial joints • Arises on disruption of the transverse ligament, and a rotatory component at the superior cervical segment is absent during flexion • May result in spinal cord injury • This condition is very rare in individuals with no predisposing factors such as Down's syndrome and rheumatoid arthritis
Hangman fracture	• A highly unstable fracture associated with the dislocation of C2–C3 facet joints • Commonly resultant of motor vehicle accidents • Bilateral fractures occur through the C2 pedicles • Incidence of 0.4 per 100,000 people

Sources: Goldberg et al. (2001); Hall et al. (2015); Hu et al. (2014); Labler et al. (2004); Lacy and Gillis (2018); Robinson et al. (2017); Standring (2016); Tenny and Varacallo (2018); Trafton (1982)

Red flags

Therapists should check for red flags (or alarm signals) that may indicate underlying pathology in patients by means of a thorough history and physical examination (Haider *et al.* 2018) (see Table 4.4). Thorough screening of a patient's examination data will help therapists to determine with a greater degree of accuracy if a patient's referral to a physician is warranted (Olson 2016). Recent guidelines outline a variety of red flags that are associated with an increased risk of the presence of serious, underlying pathology in the spine (Verhagen *et al.* 2016). When a therapist has up-to-date 'red flag' knowledge, their self-confidence takes a positive boost and this, in turn, inspires patient confidence, even when the therapist highlights signs of a serious disorder that may need further investigation (Greenhalgh and Selfe 2006). 'Most guidelines recommend screening for red flags, there is variation in which red flags are endorsed, and there exists heterogeneity in precise definitions of the red flags' (Verhagen *et al.* 2016, p.2). If a red flag symptom is detected, the therapist should use good clinical judgement and extreme caution to minimise the risk of unnecessary adverse events after CSM (see Table 4.4).

Cervical artery dysfunction covers a range of disorders that can involve the internal carotid and vertebral arteries, with dissections being the most widely reported in the literature (Buja and Butany 2016; Vaughan *et al.* 2016). The therapist needs to screen for carotid artery dissection (CAD) and vertebral artery dissection (VAD) before CSM to prevent post-manipulative adverse events (Puentedura *et al.* 2012; Vaughan *et al.* 2016). Signs associated with dissection such as headache or neck pain should not be ignored, especially since severe pain remains the hallmark for screening (Britt and Bhimji 2018; Vaughan *et al.* 2016). When screening for dissection, the therapist would do well to check the patient for a history of infection, diabetes mellitus, tobacco use or pulsating tinnitus, or physically examine for upper and lower extremity weakness, ataxia, blood pressure, proprioception and vessel palpation (Chung *et al.* 2015; Hutting *et al.* 2013; Kerry and Taylor 2014; Vaughan *et al.* 2016). The importance of proactive screening for blood pressure with regard to cervical artery dysfunction cannot be overemphasised, as this vital sign reflects the baseline cardiovascular status of the patient and guides manual therapy prescription (Frese, Fick and Sadowsky 2011). A history of trauma should strongly urge the therapist to refer for neurological imaging with CTA (computed tomography angiography) or MRI (magnetic resonance imaging) (Gross, Fetto and Rosen 2016; Vaughan *et al.* 2016).

Table 4.4. Red flags for serious pathology in the cervical spine

Condition	Incidence (estimated)	Signs and symptoms
Vertebral artery insufficiency	1 per 400,000 to 6 per 10,000,000 receiving CSM	Drop attacks Dizziness/vertigo Dysarthria Diplopia Light-headedness related to head movements Cranial nerve signs

Condition	Incidence (estimated)	Signs and symptoms
Cervical myelopathy	1.6 per 100,000 people	Sensory disturbances of the hand Wasting of intrinsic hand muscles Clonus Babinski sign Hoffman reflex Unsteady gait Disturbances of the bladder and bowel Inverted supinator sign Hyperreflexia Multi-segmental weakness or sensory changes Age >45 years
Inflammatory or systemic disease	5–7 per 100 in Western societies	Gradual onset of symptoms Family history of inflammatory disease Fatigue Temperature >37°C (100°F) Blood pressure >160/95 mmHg Resting pulse >100 bpm Resting respiration >25 bpm
Neoplastic conditions	559 per 100,000 European men and 454 per 100,000 European women	Age >50 years History of cancer Constant pain that does not subside with bed rest Unexplained weight loss Night pain
Upper cervical ligamentous instability	0.6 per 100 patients receiving chiropractic care	Post trauma Occipital headache and numbness Severe limitation during the neck's active range of motion in all directions Signs of cervical myelopathy Down's syndrome, rheumatoid arthritis
Other serious cervical pathology		Previous diagnosis of vertebrobasilar insufficiency Ataxia Nausea Dysphasia

Adapted from various sources: Boogaarts and Bartels (2015); Childs et al. (2005); El-Gabalawy, Guenther and Bernstein (2010); Hutting et al. (2013); Lestuzzi, Oliva and Ferraù (2017); Olson (2016); Puentedura et al. (2012); WHO (2005)

Special tests

Appropriate special tests for CSM can be viewed in Table 4.5. It is paramount that interpretations of special tests are reviewed frequently.

This table is not an exhaustive list of special tests but gives you, the therapist, a guide for this area. If you are unsure of the interpretation of any test that you complete with your patient, we advise that you refer to the most appropriate medical professional for further investigations.

Table 4.5. Special tests for cervical spine dysfunction

Test	Procedure	Positive sign	Interpretation
Vertebral artery test	The patient assumes either a supine lying or sitting position with the head resting on a pillow and the top of the head in line with the edge of the table. The patient must be instructed to focus on the therapist's forehead throughout the testing exercise. With the therapist supporting the patient's head, the cervical spine is slowly rotated to the right to the limit of available range. The therapist pauses for 3–5 seconds while assessing the patient's response and observing for vertebrobasilar insufficiency symptoms If a positive response is observed, the therapist must immediately reposition the head to a neutral or slightly flexed position and continue to monitor the patient Sensitivity = 0	• Faintness • Nausea and vomiting • Drop attacks • Temporary loss of hearing or vision • Pins and needles • Double vision • Sallowness and perspiration • Paralysis • Dysarthria	✓ Compression or occlusion of the vertebral artery

Test	Procedure	Positive sign	Interpretation
Sharp-Purser test	The patient's forehead is constrained posteriorly with the cranial arm in a plane parallel with the superior aspect of C2 with the caudal hand stabilising C2. If the head slides posteriorly in relation to the axis, this indicates atlantoaxial instability. The manual manoeuvre decreases the atlantoaxial subluxation that results from a semi-flexed posture in patients with atlantoaxial instability. Excessive posterior cranial glide or pain relief following the test are considered positive findings Specificity = 96% Predictive value = 85%	• Excessive posterior cranial glide, or • Pain relief following the test • A 'clunk' sound	✓ Atlantoaxial instability
Spurling's test	While the patient is seated, the therapist stands behind the patient with their hands interlocking the crown of the patient's cranium. The therapist passively side-bends the head toward the symptomatic side, applying a compressive overpressure Sensitivity = 30% Specificity = 93%	• Neck or arm symptom reproduction	✓ Foraminal encroachment
Distraction test	The patient takes a supine posture on a bed with the head relaxed on a small pillow. The therapist gently grasps the axis about its neural arch with one hand while holding the occiput with the other. The therapist then flexes the patient's neck to a comfortable position by elevating the head approximately 20–25° from the horizontal plane. A distraction force of up to 14 kg is gradually applied. If no symptoms are observed in the neutral plane, the test ought to be done again in slight flexion and then extension Specificity = 94% Sensitivity = 44%	• Excessive vertical translation when manual traction is applied • Reduction of symptoms with application of cervical distraction force	✓ Tectorial membrane instability ✓ Upper cervical ligamentous instability

Sources: Grant (1996); Hartley (1995); Mintken, Metrick and Flynn (2008); Olson (2016); Osmotherly, Rivett and Rowe (2012); Rubinstein et al. (2007)

References

Boogaarts, H.D. and Bartels, R.H.M.A. (2015) 'Prevalence of cervical spondylotic myelopathy.' *European Spine Journal* 24(S2), 139–141. doi:10.1007/s00586-013-2781-x

Britt, T.B. and Bhimji, S.S. (2018) 'Vertebral artery dissection.' *StatPearls*. Available at www.ncbi. nlm.nih.gov/pubmed/28722857

Bronfort, G., Evans, R., Anderson, A.V., Svendsen, K.H., Bracha, Y. and Grimm, R.H. (2012) 'Spinal manipulation, medication, or home exercise with advice for acute and subacute neck pain.' *Annals of Internal Medicine* 156(Part 1), 1. doi:10.7326/0003-4819-156-1-201201030-00002

Budd, M.A., Hough, S., Wegener, S.T. and Stiers, W. (2017) *Practical Psychology in Medical Rehabilitation*. Cham, Switzerland: Springer. doi:10.1007/978-3-319-34034-0

Buja, L.M. and Butany, J. (2016) *Cardiovascular Pathology*. Amsterdam: Elsevier.

Cassidy, J.D., Boyle, E., Côté, P., He, Y., Hogg-Johnson, S., Silver, F.L. *et al.* (2008) 'Risk of vertebrobasilar stroke and chiropractic care.' *Spine* 33(Supplement), S176–S183. doi:10.1097/BRS.0b013e3181644600

Childs, J.D., Flynn, T.W., Fritz, J.M., Piva, S.R., Whitman, J.M., Wainner, R.S. *et al.* (2005) 'Screening for vertebrobasilar insufficiency in patients with neck pain: Manual therapy decision-making in the presence of uncertainty.' *Journal of Orthopaedic & Sports Physical Therapy* 35(5), 300–306. Available at www.ncbi.nlm.nih.gov/pubmed/15966541

Chung, C.L., Côté, P., Stern, P. and L'Espérance, G. (2015) 'The association between cervical spine manipulation and carotid artery dissection: A systematic review of the literature.' *Journal of Manipulative and Physiological Therapeutics* 38(9), 672–676. doi:10.1016/j.jmpt.2013.09.005

El-Gabalawy, H., Guenther, L.C. and Bernstein, C.N. (2010) 'Epidemiology of immune-mediated inflammatory diseases: Incidence, prevalence, natural history, and comorbidities.' *Journal of Rheumatology* 37(Suppl. 85), 2–10. doi:10.3899/jrheum.091461

Ernst, E. (2007) 'Adverse effects of spinal manipulation: A systematic review.' *Journal of the Royal Society of Medicine* 100(7), 330–338. doi:10.1258/jrsm.100.7.330

Frese, E.M., Fick, A. and Sadowsky, H.S. (2011) 'Blood pressure measurement guidelines for physical therapists.' *Cardiopulmonary Physical Therapy Journal* 22(2), 5–12. Available at www.ncbi.nlm.nih.gov/pubmed/21637392

Goldberg, W., Mueller, C., Panacek, E., Tigges, S., Hoffman, J.R., Mower, W.R. *et al.* (2001) 'Distribution and patterns of blunt traumatic cervical spine injury.' *Annals of Emergency Medicine* 38(1), 17–21. doi:10.1067/mem.2001.116150

Grant, R. (1996) 'Vertebral artery testing – The Australian Physiotherapy Association Protocol after 6 years.' *Manual Therapy* 1(3), 149–153. doi:10.1016/S0039-6109(16)42634-4

Greenhalgh, S. and Selfe, J. (2006) *Red Flags: A Guide to Identifying Serious Pathology of the Spine*. Philadelphia, PA: Churchill Livingstone Elsevier.

Gross, J.M., Fetto, J. and Rosen, E. (2016) *Musculoskeletal Examination*. 4th edn. Chichester: John Wiley & Sons.

Haider, Z., Rossiter, D., Shafafy, R., Kieffer, W. and Thomas, M. (2018) 'How not to miss major spinal pathology in neck pain.' *British Journal of Hospital Medicine* 79(7), C98–C102. doi:10.12968/hmed.2018.79.7.C98

Hall, G.C., Kinsman, M.J., Nazar, R.G., Hruska, R.T., Mansfield, K.J., Boakye, M., *et al.* (2015) 'Atlanto-occipital dislocation.' *World Journal of Orthopedics* 6(2), 236–243. doi:10.5312/wjo.v6.i2.236

Hartley, A. (1995) *Practical Joint Assessment: Upper Quadrant: A Sports Medicine Manual*. St Louis, MO: Mosby.

Hu, Y., Albert, T.J., Kepler, C.K., Ma, W.-H., Yuan, Z.-S. and Dong, W.-X. (2014) 'Unstable Jefferson fractures: Results of transoral osteosynthesis.' *Indian Journal of Orthopaedics* 48(2), 145–151. doi:10.4103/0019-5413.128750

Hutting, N., Scholten-Peeters, G.G.M., Vijverman, V., Keesenberg, M.D.M. and Verhagen, A.P. (2013) 'Diagnostic accuracy of upper cervical spine instability tests: A systematic review.' *Physical Therapy* 93(12), 1686–1695. doi:10.2522/ptj.20130186

Hutting, N., Kerry, R., Coppieters, M.W. and Scholten-Peeters, G.G.M. (2018) 'Considerations to improve the safety of cervical spine manual therapy.' *Musculoskeletal Science and Practice* 33, 41–45. doi:10.1016/j.msksp.2017.11.003

Johnson, R. (1991) 'Anatomy of the Cervical Spine and its Related Structures.' In J. Torg (ed.) *Athletic Injuries to the Head, Neck, and Face.* St Louis, MO: Mosby.

Kennell, K.A., Daghfal, M.M., Patel, S.G., SeSanto, J.R., Waterman, G.S. and Bertino, R.E. (2017) 'Cervical artery dissection related to chiropractic manipulation: One institution's experience.' *The Journal of Family Practice* 66(9), 556–562.

Kerry, R. and Taylor, A.J. (2014) 'Cervical spine pre-treatment screening for arterial dysfunction: Out with the old, in with the new.' *In Touch* 147(July), 10–14. doi:10.13140/2.1.1509.9526

König, A. and Spetzger, U. (2016) *Degenerative Diseases of the Cervical Spine: Therapeutic Management in the Subaxial Section.* Cham, Switzerland: Springer International Publishing. doi:10.1007/978-3-319-47298-0

Labler, L., Eid, K., Platz, A., Trentz, O. and Kossmann, T. (2004) 'Atlanto-occipital dislocation: Four case reports of survival in adults and review of the literature.' *European Spine Journal* 13(2), 172–180. doi:10.1007/s00586-003-0653-5

Lacy, J. and Gillis, C.C. (2018) 'Atlantoaxial instability.' *StatPearls.* Available at www.ncbi.nlm. nih.gov/pubmed/30137847

Lestuzzi, C., Oliva, S. and Ferraù, F. (eds) (2017) *Manual of Cardio-Oncology.* Cham, Switzerland: Springer International Publishing. doi:10.1007/978-3-319-40236-9

Mintken, P.E., Metrick, L. and Flynn, T. (2008) 'Upper cervical ligament testing in a patient with os odontoideum presenting with headaches.' *Journal of Orthopaedic & Sports Physical Therapy* 38(8), 465–475. doi:10.2519/jospt.2008.2747

Olson, K.A. (2016) *Manual Physical Therapy of the Spine.* 2nd edn. St Louis, MO: Elsevier.

Osmotherly, P.G., Rivett, D.A. and Rowe, L.J. (2012) 'The anterior shear and distraction tests for craniocervical instability. An evaluation using magnetic resonance imaging.' *Manual Therapy* 17(5), 416–421. doi:10.1016/j.math.2012.03.010

Puentedura, E.J., March, J., Anders, J., Perez, A., Landers, M.R., Wallmann, H.W. *et al.* (2012) 'Safety of cervical spine manipulation: Are adverse events preventable and are manipulations being performed appropriately? A review of 134 case reports.' *The Journal of Manual and Manipulative Therapy* 20(2), 66–74. doi:10.1179/2042618611Y.0000000022

Robinson, A.-L., Möller, A., Robinson, Y. and Olerud, C. (2017) 'C2 fracture subtypes, incidence, and treatment allocation change with age: A retrospective cohort study of 233 consecutive cases.' *BioMed Research International*, 1–7. doi:10.1155/2017/8321680

Rubinstein, S.M., Pool, J.J., van Tulder, M.W., Riphagen, I.I. and de Vet, H.C. (2007) 'A systematic review of the diagnostic accuracy of provocative tests of the neck for diagnosing cervical radiculopathy.' *European Spine Journal* 16(3), 307–319. doi:10.1007/s00586-006-0225-6

Rushton, A., Rivett, D., Carlesso, L., Flynn, T., Hing, W. and Kerry, R. (2014) 'International framework for examination of the cervical region for potential of cervical arterial dysfunction prior to orthopaedic manual therapy intervention.' *Manual Therapy* 19(3), 222–228. doi:10.1016/j.math.2013.11.005

Schafer, R.C. and Faye, L. (1990) *Motion Palpation and Chiropractic Technic: Principles of Dynamic Chiropractic.* Huntington Beach, CA: Motion Palpation Institute.

Shen, F.H., Samartzis, D. and Fessler, R.G. (eds) (2015) *Textbook of the Cervical Spine.* St Louis, MO: Elsevier Inc. Available at http://link.springer.com/10.1007/978-3-319-47298-0

Souza, T.A. (2016) *Differential Diagnosis and Management for the Chiropractor: Protocols and Algorithms.* 5th edn. Burlington, VA: Jones & Bartlett Learning.

Standring, S. (ed.) (2016) *Gray's Anatomy: The Anatomical Basis of Clinical Practice.* 41st edn. New York: Elsevier. Available at www.elsevier.com/books/grays-anatomy/standring/978-0-7020-5230-9

Tenny, S. and Varacallo, M. (2018) 'Fracture, odontoid.' *StatPearls*. Available at www.ncbi.nlm. nih.gov/pubmed/28722985

Trafton, P.G. (1982) 'Spinal cord injuries.' *Surgical Clinics of North America* 62(1), 61–72. doi:10.1016/S0039-6109(16)42634-4

Tubbs, R.S., Dixon, J., Loukas, M., Shoja, M.M. and Cohen-Gadol, A.A. (2010) 'Ligament of Barkow of the craniocervical junction: Its anatomy and potential clinical and functional significance.' *Journal of Neurosurgery: Spine* 12(6), 619–622. doi:10.3171/2009.12.SPINE09671

Tubbs, R.S., Hallock, J.D., Radcliff, V., Naftel, R.P., Mortazavi, M., Shoja, M.M. *et al.* (2011) 'Ligaments of the craniocervical junction.' *Journal of Neurosurgery: Spine* 14(6), 697–709. doi:10.3171/2011.1.SPINE10612

Vaughan, B., Moran, R., Tehan, P., Fryer, G., Holmes, M., Vogel, S. *et al.* (2016) 'Manual therapy and cervical artery dysfunction: Identification of potential risk factors in clinical encounters.' *International Journal of Osteopathic Medicine* 21, 40–50. doi:10.1016/j.ijosm.2016.01.007

Verhagen, A.P., Downie, A., Popal, N., Maher, C. and Koes, B.W. (2016) 'Red flags presented in current low back pain guidelines: A review.' *European Spine Journal* 25(9), 2788–2802. doi:10.1007/s00586-016-4684-0

White, A.A. and Panjabi, M.M. (1990) *Clinical Biomechanics of the Spine*. Philadelphia, PA: Lippincott.

WHO (World Health Organization) (2005) *WHO Guidelines on Basic Training and Safety in Chiropractic*. Geneva: WHO.

Yamamoto, K., Condotta, L., Haldane, C., Jaffrani, S., Johnstone, V., Jachyra, P. *et al.* (2018) 'Exploring the teaching and learning of clinical reasoning, risks, and benefits of cervical spine manipulation.' *Physiotherapy Theory and Practice* 34(2), 91–100. doi:10.1080/09593985.201 7.1375056

CERVICAL SPINE MANIPULATION TECHNIQUES

Seated C2-C7 manipulation

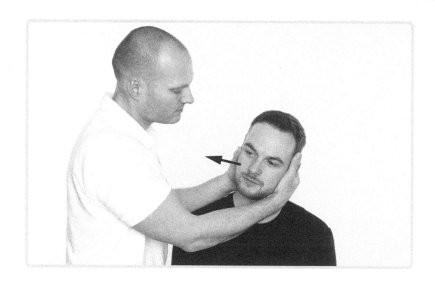

- Stand to the side to which you will rotate the patient's head, with the patient sitting comfortably.

- With your contact hand, locate the chosen segment articular pillar, counting down from C2 spinous process (SP).

- Finish with your 2nd and 3rd finger at the desired spinal segment to manipulate.

- Apply the support hand under the occipital area.

- Ask the patient to relax their head into your contact hand. Control their head into flexion and side-bending.

- Side-bend towards the contact hand and simultaneously rotate away, maintaining neck flexion.

- Optimise this movement, keeping your elbows in close to your body.

- Engage the barrier where the pivot point is directly over your contact hand.

- Ask the patient to inhale and exhale.

- Apply the manipulation at the end of exhalation.

Recumbent C2-C7 manipulation

- Stand to the side to which you will rotate the patient's head, with the patient in a recumbent position.

- With your contact hand, locate the chosen segment articular pillar, counting down from C2 SP.

- Finish with your 2nd and 3rd finger at the desired spinal segment to manipulate.

- Apply the support hand under the occipital area.

- Ask the patient to relax their head into your contact hand. Control their head into flexion and side-bending.

- Side-bend towards the contact hand and simultaneously rotate away, maintaining neck flexion.

- Optimise this movement, keeping your elbows in close to your body.

- Engage the barrier where the pivot point is directly over your contact hand.

- Ask the patient to inhale and exhale.

- Apply the manipulation at the end of exhalation.

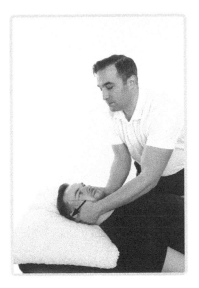

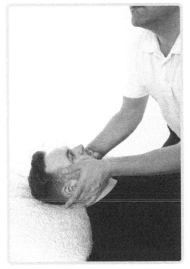

Prone C2-C7 manipulation

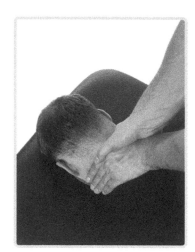

- The patient is prone, with the therapist standing to the side of the table.

- To set up for the prone oblique thrust, with your dominant hand, locate the chosen segment articular pillar, counting down from C2 SP, and contact with your first metacarpal phalangeal joint (MCP). Only apply light pressure, ensuring the fingers don't grip the lateral aspect of the neck.

- With the other hand, reinforce the contact hand to ensure you are supporting and protecting your fingers.

- Apply gentle pressure towards the target segment in an inferior oblique angle, taking up the tissue slack to build pre-tension.

- Ask the patient to relax their head.

- Using the contact hand, apply an oblique drive inferior, aiming towards the nose or the face hole of the table.

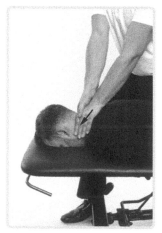
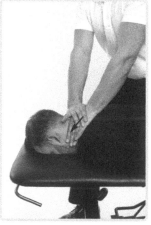
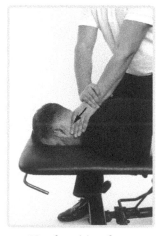

Hand position one, reinforced thumb contact over target segment

Hand position two, reinforced finger contact over target segment

Hand position three, reinforced wrist

Side-lying C2-C7 manipulation

- The patient is in a side-lying position, with the therapist standing to the side of the table.

- With your contact hand, locate the chosen segment articular pillar, counting down from C2 SP.

- Finish with your 2nd and 3rd finger at the desired spinal segment to manipulate.

- Apply the other hand under the occipital area.

- Ask the patient to relax their head into your contact hand. Control their head into flexion and side-bending.

- Side-bend towards the contact hand and simultaneously rotate away, maintaining neck flexion.

- Optimise this movement, keeping your elbows in close to your body.

- Engage the barrier where the pivot point is directly over your contact hand.

- Ask the patient to inhale and exhale.

- Apply the manipulation at the end of exhalation.

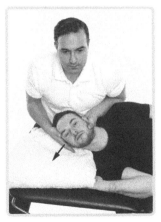 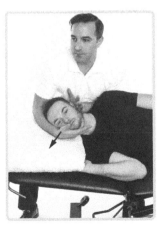 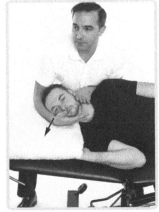

Hand position one,
thumb contact

Hand position two,
pisiform contact

Hand position three,
MCP contact

Side-lying occipital-atlantal and atlantal-axial (OA-AA) manipulation

- Fully rotate the patient's head and then bring it back halfway to 50% of rotation.

- With your contact hand, locate the base of the ipsilateral occiput, atlas or transverse process (TVP) of C2.

- Your support hand should gently cradle the contra-lateral occipital area.

- Using the thenar eminence of your contact hand, contact over the zygomatic arch, maintaining a light contact.

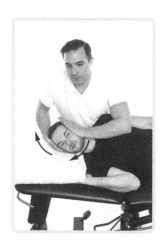

- Keeping the weight of the patient's head on the pillow, begin to side-bend the patient's head over your point of contact.

- To help with this movement, shift your body towards the side of the contact hand, keeping relaxed, bent knees in a lunge movement.

- Keeping your elbow tucked in, ensure your arm is positioned in the direction of the line of drive.

- The line of drive should be directly through the opposite occiput into side-bending, with moderate traction from the support hand.

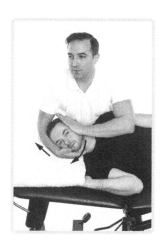

Hand position two

- For C1/C2, the line of drive can be slightly more rotary and directed slightly lower to affect the desired segment.

- Engage the barrier.

- Ask the patient to inhale and exhale.

The alternative hand position is to use a chin grip technique instead of a sub-occipital hold. This allows you to bring the patient's head into full side-bending while applying contact over the zygomatic arch.

Seated OA-AA manipulation

- The patient is in a seated position, with the therapist standing to the side of them.

- Apply contact against the patient's temple with your sternum, to apply counter-pressure.

- With your contact hand, locate the base of the contra-lateral occiput, atlas or TVP of C2. The contact will be on the mastoid process with a reinforced supporting hand contact.

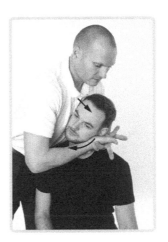

- Your support hand should gently cradle the contra-lateral occipital area.

- Get the patient to drop the shoulder on the contact side to help take out any tissue slack, maintaining a light contact.

- As the patient drops their shoulder on the contra-lateral side, apply side-bending pressure via your sternum while your hands produce a 'J' movement towards you.

- Engage the barrier.

- Ask the patient to inhale and exhale.

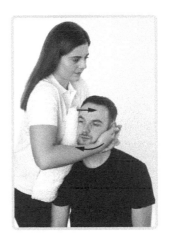

Hand position two

- The line of drive should be directly through the opposite occiput into side-bending, with moderate traction from the support hand.

An alternative technique for female patients is to use a towel to create a barrier between your sternum and the patient's temple.

Prone OA-AA manipulation

- The patient is in a prone position, with the therapist standing at the head of the table.

- Rest the patient's head on the forearm of your contact hand, and locate the base of the contra-lateral occiput, atlas or TVP of C2. The supporting arm will contact the temple with the supporting hand sitting below the cervico-thoracic junction (CTJ).

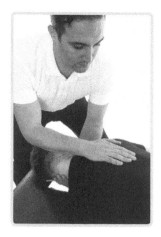

- Your support hand should gently cradle the contra-lateral occipital area, and the patient's chin should rest on your forearm comfortably, maintaining a light contact.

- Stabilising the patient's head, apply a side-bending pressure with the uppermost arm.

- Engage the barrier.

- Ask the patient to inhale and exhale.

- The line of drive should be directly through the opposite occiput into side-bending, with moderate traction from the support hand.

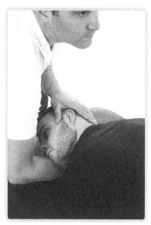

Hand position two

An alternative hand position is with the supporting hand contacting the temporalis and sub-occipital ridge.

TEMPOROMANDIBULAR JOINT (TMJ) MANIPULATION TECHNIQUES

TMJ thumb and chin-hold manipulation

- The patient lies down in the supine position with the head in slight flexion and rotation (use a towel or pillow).

- Stand in an asymmetrical stance (outside leg facing forwards), facing the patient.

- Your left hand palpates over the left masseter while your 1st MCP prevents the neck from moving into extension.

- Your right hand loosely holds the patient's chin.

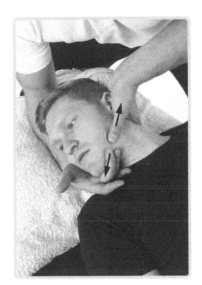

- To engage the barrier, the patient relaxes their jaw while your left thumb places pressure back towards you and downwards towards the TMJ.

- Your right hand adds pressure towards the jaw inferiorly.

- Ask the patient to breathe in and out.

- On the breath out, simultaneously perform your manipulation from both hands, as shown.

Key to note:

- Make sure the patient relaxes their jaw.

- Wait until the last second to fully engage the barrier.

- Avoid placing too much pressure over the masseter.

- Avoid this technique if there is significant history of dislocation.

TMJ chin contact

- The patient lies down in the supine position with the head in slight flexion and rotation (use a towel or pillow).

- Stand in an asymmetrical stance (outside leg facing forwards), facing the patient.

- Place your 1st MCP into the lamina groove and locate the affected TMJ with your thumb.

- The thumb on the affected side aids the stabilisation of the technique while allowing accurate palpation of the joint line.

- Your right hand supports the head and contacts the mandible.

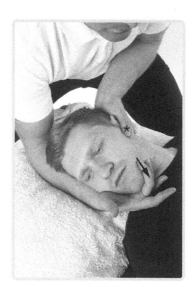

- To engage the barrier, stabilise the affected TMJ and ask the patient to breathe in and out.

- As they are completing their expiration, perform your manipulation with the line of drive down the line of the mandible.

Key to note:

- Avoid the temptation to add too much rotation as this will focus the force of the manipulation on the cervical spine.

- Avoid this technique if there is significant history of dislocation.

TMJ manipulation using pisiform or thenar eminence

- The patient lies down in the supine position with the head in slight flexion and rotation (use a towel or pillow).

- Stand in an asymmetrical stance (outside leg facing forwards), facing the patient.

- Either stabilise the head from the contra-lateral mastoid process (first picture) or the ipsilateral temporalis (second picture).

- Contact the mandible either on the mandibular angle (first picture) or along the mandibular line.

- The patient relaxes their jaw and is asked to breathe in and out to help.

- As they breathe out, engage the barrier with pressure along the mandibular angle and perform your manipulation.

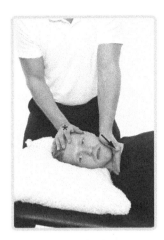

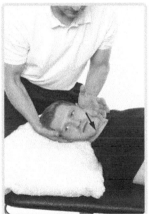

Key to note:

- Avoid the temptation to add too much rotation as this will focus the force of the manipulation on the cervical spine.

- This technique can be completed without rotation, as shown in the third picture.

- Avoid this technique if there is significant history of dislocation.

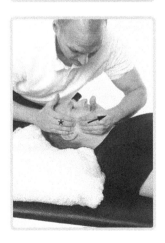

TMJ manipulation using reinforced thenar eminence

- The patient lies down in the supine position with the head in slight flexion and rotation (use a towel or pillow).

- Stand in an asymmetrical stance (outside leg facing forwards), facing the patient.

- Contact the mandible, along the mandibular line, with the thenar eminence of your hand, reinforced as shown.

- The patient relaxes their jaw and is asked to breathe in and out to help.

- As they breathe out, engage the barrier with pressure along the mandibular angle and perform your manipulation.

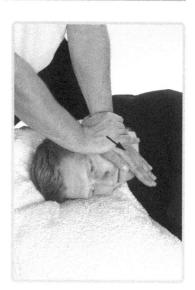

Key to note:

- Avoid the temptation to add too much rotation as this will focus the force of the manipulation on the cervical spine.

- Avoid crossing the patient's face to complete this manipulation.

- Avoid this technique if there is significant history of dislocation.

5

THE THORACIC SPINE

Introduction

The thoracic spine is an important target for manipulative therapy as a relatively greater number of patients receive thoracic spine manipulation (TSM) compared with other spinal regions (Heneghan *et al.* 2018; Thornton 2018). A variety of manipulation techniques can be employed at the different segments of the thoracic spine to alleviate pain and increase mobility in patients (Ditcharles *et al.* 2017). Therapists often use thrust (high-velocity, low-amplitude (HVLA) force) or non-thrust (cyclic low-velocity force) manipulation of the thoracic region to treat various thoracic and cervical spine conditions among other maladies (Griswold *et al.* 2018; Puentedura and O'Grady 2015).

The benefits of TSM apply to a variety of orthopaedic conditions as thoracic spine function is key to preserving health for various locations on the axial skeleton (Howe and Read 2015). A study by Rhon, Greenlee and Fritz (2018) reported that TSM was the most frequently utilised form of manipulation for patients with thoracic conditions, with over 50 per cent of individuals receiving this form of therapy. Masaracchio *et al.* (2019) also reported TSM to be beneficial for the management of individuals suffering from mechanical neck pain. These studies, while outlining some direct benefits of TSM in specific patient conditions, also demonstrate the promise of TSM as an ideal non-invasive treatment modality. A word of caution from Puentedura and O'Grady (2015), however, warns therapists against using excessive peak forces in TSM as this may result in unintended adverse effects.

This chapter outlines some key concepts for the therapist seeking to utilise TSM such as common injuries of the thoracic spine, red flags for potentially serious pathology and special diagnostic tests appropriate to this spinal region. As a primer to the outlined concepts, the chapter also includes an overview of various thoracic joints as well as their ranges of motion.

Joints

The thoracic spine attaches to the cervical spine superiorly and to the lumbar spine inferiorly. It consists of 12 vertebrae, numbered T1–T12 (see Table 5.1). The vertebrae caudally increase in size, towards the lumbar spine (Liebsch and Wilke 2018). The spines form various joints that are classified into two categories: those that are found throughout the vertebral column and those exclusive to the thoracic spine. Those joints unique to the thoracic spine include the costovertebral and costotransverse forming articulations with the ribs and the zygapophysial joints (Wilke *et al.* 2017).

Table 5.1. Joints of the thoracic spine

Joint name	Description	Function
Costovertebral joint	• This is a gliding joint • Forms a juncture at which the head of a rib articulates with the vertebral body of a thoracic vertebra • Supported by various ligaments including radiate, costotransverse, lateral costotransverse and superior costotransverse ligaments	• Plays a role in thoracic stabilisation, load bearing, protection and mobility • Helps support spinal movement • Enables respiratory movement of the chest wall • Allows slight gliding movements
Costotransverse joint	• The point at which the neck and tubercle of a given rib are united with the transverse process of its corresponding thoracic vertebra • Consists of medial and lateral facets • Medial facet forms a synovial joint with the tip of the transverse process which is reinforced by a capsule • Lateral facet is attached to the transverse process through ligaments • Strengthened by lateral costotransverse, costotransverse and superior costotransverse ligaments • Consists of a capsule, the neck and tubercle ligaments and costotransverse ligaments • The synovial joint is present in all vertebrae except T11 and T12	• Allows slight medial and lateral-oriented gliding movements of the ribs
Zygapophysial joints (facet joints)	• A diarthrodial joint • A set of two synovial joints in each spinal motion segment • Formed between the superior articular process and the inferior articular process of adjacent vertebrae • Positioned vertically	• Offers structural stability to the vertebral column • Limits flexion and extension • Facilitates rotation • Guides and constrains the motion of the vertebrae

Sources: Liebsch and Wilke (2018); Saker et al. (2016); Wilke et al. (2017)

Range of motion

The thoracic spine possesses the least range of motion in comparison with the cervical and lumbar spine (see Table 5.2). This distinction is attributable to the articulations with the rib cage and the orientation of the facets (Liebsch and Wilke 2018). Both the range of motion and the neutral zone decreases inferiorly for equal bending moments (Hajibozorgi and Arjmand 2016; Wilke *et al.* 2017).

Table 5.2. Range of motion between different thoracic joints

Movement	Motion unit	Range of motion
Flexion	C7–T1	9° (approximately)
	T1–T6	4°
	T6–T7	4–8°
	T12–L1	8–12°
Lateral bending	T1–T10	6° (approximately)
	T11–L1	8° (approximately)
Sagittal	T1–T10	Less than 5°
	T10–T12	5° (approximately)
Rotation	T1–T4	8–12°
	T5–T8	8° (approximately)
	T9–T12	Less than 3°

Sources: McKenzie and May (2006); Page et al. (2018)

Common injuries

Injuries to the thoracic spine (see Table 5.3) have a lower incidence compared with the cervical and lumbar spine, due to amplified biomechanical support (Liebsch and Wilke 2018; Menzer, Gill and Paterson 2015). However, when a thoracic injury occurs, the effects are greatly feared due to the potential for a disastrous neurological complication (Menzer *et al.* 2015). An injury to the thoracic spine may be due to an accident in aggressive sports using the upper extremities, falls, violent activity or road traffic accident (Wilke *et al.* 2017). Owing to the infrequent occurrence of injuries, diagnosis and treatment have been reported to not be very easy (Menzer *et al.* 2015). Injuries usually result in a fracture in the thoracic vertebra, and subsequently to pain and poor spinal functioning depending on the severity (Liebsch and Wilke 2018).

Table 5.3. Common injuries of the thoracic joints

Common injuries	Incidence	Characteristics
Compression fracture	• 10.7 per 1000 person-years in women (EU) • 5.7 per 1000 person-years in men (EU) • 123 per 100,000 person-years (USA)	• Occurs when a bone in the spine anteriorly collapses, usually T11, T12 and L1 • Usually a stable fracture, as it doesn't move the bones out of their positions • Does not lead to neurological complications • Prevalent in osteoporosis patients, hard falls, excessive pressure or physical injury
Vertebral body fracture	• Not reported	• Prevalent in the thoracolumbar region • Frequently results from a high-energy accident or osteoporosis • Common in people with ankylosing spondylitis, a vertebral tumour or infection • Indications include pain or the development of neural deficits such as numbness, weakness, tingling, spinal shock or neurogenic shock • Principally occurs more in men than in women
Fracture dislocation	• 1.6 per million (USA) • 0.52 per million (Ireland)	• Caused by high-energy force • Common in patients with polytrauma • The injury results in thoracic vertebra fractures and moves off an adjacent vertebra • Often accompanied by neurological symptoms
Transverse process fracture	• Not reported	• Due to various causes such as blunt trauma, violent lateral flexion-extension forces • Frequently occurs due to a direct blow to the thoracic region such as a gun shot • Spinal cord stability is not usually affected

Sources: EPOS Group et al. (2002); Jiang et al. (2014); Mathis et al. (2001); Newell et al. (2018); Singh et al. (2014); Watts (2016)

Red flags

Red flag symptoms are useful for identifying potentially serious pathology in patients reporting thoracic pain. When any of the red flag symptoms outlined in Table 5.4 are found or suspected in a patient, the therapist should use sound clinical judgement and make cautious decisions so as to minimise the risk of adverse events resulting from TSM (WHO 2005).

Table 5.4. Red flags for serious pathology in the thoracic spine

Condition	Signs and symptoms
Spinal tumours	<ul><li>Age >50 years</li><li>History of malignancy</li><li>Unplanned weight loss</li><li>Relentless and progressive pain at night</li><li>Pain for over a month</li><li>No recovery with standard treatment</li></ul>
Spinal infection	<ul><li>Age >50 years</li><li>Recent incidence of bacterial infection (e.g., tuberculosis, urinary tract infection, skin infection)</li><li>Intravenous drug use</li><li>Relentless fever or systemic disease</li></ul>
Spinal cord lesion	<ul><li>Bowel or bladder dysfunction</li><li>Positive extensor plantar response</li><li>Increased muscle tone, muscle spasticity, hyperreflexia or clonus</li><li>Motor weakness, loss of dexterity, disturbed gait, clumsiness</li><li>Extensive paraesthesia</li></ul>
Fracture	<ul><li>Age >70 years</li><li>Recent history of major trauma</li><li>Corticosteroid use</li><li>History of osteoporosis</li></ul>
Inflammatory arthropathy	<ul><li>Steady onset beginning before 40 years of age</li><li>Family history of arthropathy</li><li>Noticeable morning stiffness</li><li>Continuous restriction of movement</li><li>Peripheral joints involved</li><li>Discharge from the urethra, iritis or colitis, or skin rash</li></ul>
Vascular/ neurological	<ul><li>Intense light-headedness</li><li>Episodes of collapsing or loss of consciousness</li><li>Positive cranial nerve signs</li></ul>

Sources: Lake et al. (2018); Magee (2014); McKenzie and May (2006)

Special tests

Table 5.5 is not an exhaustive list of special tests but gives you, the therapist, a guide for this area. If you are unsure of the interpretation of any test that you complete with your patient, we advise that you refer to the most appropriate medical professional for further investigations.

Table 5.5. Special tests for thoracic spine dysfunction

Test	Procedure	Positive sign	Interpretation	Test statistics
Cervical rotation lateral flexion test	The test is conducted with the patient seated. The therapist, standing behind the patient, passively and maximally rotates the head away from the painful side. The therapist gently flexes the head laterally, as far as possible	• Lateral flexion movement is blocked	✓ First rib hypomobility in patients with brachialgia	Specificity: Not reported Sensitivity: Not reported
Passive rotation test	The patient is seated with their hands clasped behind their neck. The therapist uses their thumb and index finger to palpate both sides of a spinous process, just lateral to the interspinous space. The therapist rotates the patient's shoulders either rightward or leftward, comparing the amount and quality of segmental movement by palpation	• Hard end-feel • Empty end-feel often accompanied by muscle spasm • Heightened pain with head movement	✓ A hard end-feel is often suggestive of ankylosing spondylitis or advanced arthrosis ✓ An empty end-feel with muscle spasm is suggestive of a severe disorder (e.g., neoplasm) ✓ Increased pain with head movement is a dural sign	Specificity: Not reported Sensitivity: Not reported

Test	Procedure	Positive sign	Interpretation	Test statistics
Anterior-posterior rib compression test	The test is conducted with the patient seated or standing. The therapist stands or crouches behind the patient and places their arms around the patient's chest, applying sagittal and horizontal compressional force	• Rib shaft prominence in midaxillary line • Localised pain or point tenderness with ribcage compression • Inspiration and expiration limitations	✓ Possible rib fracture, costochondral separation or contusion ✓ Motion restriction or irritation in the sternocostal, costotransverse or costovertebral joints	Specificity: Not reported Sensitivity: Not reported
Brudzinski–Kernig test	In the Brudzinski part of the test, the patient assumes a supine posture on the table. The therapist then elevates the patient's head from the table, while restraining the upper body In the Kernig portion, the patient, lying supine, flexes both hips and knees at 90°. The patient then extends the flexed knee	• Brudzinski – involuntary flexion of the knees and hips, pulling both legs toward the chest • Kernig – patient resists full extension of the knee with complaints of pain in the lower back, neck or head	✓ Meningeal inflammation or irritation	Specificity: 0.98 Sensitivity: 0.03–0.15

Sources: Boissonnault (2005); Buckup and Buckup (2016); Dhatt and Prabhakar (2019); Douglas, Nicol and Robertson (2013); Lindgren, Leino and Manninen (1992); Magee (2014); McBride et al. (2017); McGee (2017); Ombregt (2013); Starkey and Brown (2010)

References

Boissonnault, W.G. (2005) *Primary Care for the Physical Therapist*. St Louis, MO: Elsevier Saunders. doi:10.1016/B978-0-7216-9659-1.X5001-1

Buckup, K. and Buckup, J. (2016) *Clinical Tests for the Musculoskeletal System: Examinations, Signs, Phenomena*. 3rd edn. Stuttgart: Thieme Medical Publishers.

Dhatt, S.S. and Prabhakar, S. (eds) (2019) *Handbook of Clinical Examination in Orthopedics*. Singapore: Springer Singapore. doi:10.1007/978-981-13-1235-9

Ditcharles, S., Yiou, E., Delafontaine, A. and Hamaoui, A. (2017) 'Short-term effects of thoracic spine manipulation on the biomechanical organisation of gait initiation: A randomized pilot study.' *Frontiers in Human Neuroscience* 11. doi:10.3389/fnhum.2017.00343

Douglas, G., Nicol, F. and Robertson, C. (eds) (2013) *Macleod's Clinical Examination*. 13th edn. London: Churchill Livingstone Elsevier.

EPOS (European Prospective Osteoporosis Study) Group, Felsenberg, D., Silman, A.J., Lunt, M., Armbrecht, G., Ismail, A.A. *et al.* (2002) 'Incidence of vertebral fracture in Europe: Results from the European Prospective Osteoporosis Study (EPOS).' *The Journal of Bone and Mineral Research* 17(4), 716–724. doi:10.1359/jbmr.2002.17.4.716

Griswold, D., Learman, K., Kolber, M.J., O'Halloran, B. and Cleland, J.A. (2018) 'Pragmatically applied cervical and thoracic nonthrust manipulation versus thrust manipulation for patients with mechanical neck pain: A multicenter randomized clinical trial.' *Journal of Orthopaedic & Sports Physical Therapy* 48(3), 137–145. doi:10.2519/jospt.2018.7738

Hajibozorgi, M. and Arjmand, N. (2016) 'Sagittal range of motion of the thoracic spine using inertial tracking device and effect of measurement errors on model predictions.' *Journal of Biomechanics* 49(6), 913–918. doi:10.1016/j.jbiomech.2015.09.003

Heneghan, N.R., Davies, S.E., Puentedura, E.J. and Rushton, A. (2018) 'Knowledge and pre-thoracic spinal thrust manipulation examination: A survey of current practice in the UK.' *Journal of Manual & Manipulative Therapy* 26(5), 301–309. doi:10.1080/10669817.2018.1507269

Howe, L. and Read, P. (2015) 'Thoracic spine function assessment and self-management.' *Strength and Conditioning Journal* 39, 21–30.

Jiang, B., Zhu, R., Cao, Q. and Pan, H. (2014) 'Severe thoracic spinal fracture-dislocation without neurological symptoms and costal fractures: A case report and review of the literature.' *Journal of Medical Case Reports* 8(1), 343. doi:10.1186/1752-1947-8-343

Lake, C., Templin, K., Vallely Farrell, A., Lowe, R. and Prudden, G. (2018) 'Thoracic Examination.' *Physiopedia*. Available at www.physio-pedia.com/index.php?title=Thoracic_Examination&oldid=197091

Liebsch, C. and Wilke, H.-J. (2018) 'Basic Biomechanics of the Thoracic Spine and Rib Cage.' In F. Galbusera and H.-J. Wilke (eds) *Biomechanics of the Spine: Basic Concepts, Spinal Disorders and Treatments*. London: Academic Press. doi:10.1016/b978-0-12-812851-0.00003-3

Lindgren, K.-A., Leino, E. and Manninen, H. (1992) 'Cervical rotation lateral flexion test in brachialgia.' *Archives of Physical Medicine and Rehabilitation* 73(8), 735–737. doi:10.5555/URI:PII:000399939290208E

Magee, D.J. (2014) *Orthopedic Physical Assessment*. 6th edn. St Louis, MO: Saunders.

Masaracchio, M., Kirker, K., States, R., Hanney, W.J., Liu, X. and Kolber, M. (2019) 'Thoracic spine manipulation for the management of mechanical neck pain: A systematic review and meta-analysis.' *PLOS One* 14(2), e0211877. doi:10.1371/journal.pone.0211877

Mathis, J.M., Barr, J.D., Belkoff, S.M., Barr, M.S., Jensen, M.E. and Deramond, H. (2001) 'Percutaneous vertebroplasty: A developing standard of care for vertebral compression fractures.' *American Journal of Neuroradiology*. Available at www.ajnr.org/content/ajnr/22/2/373.full.pdf

McBride, S., Thomas, E., Ritchie, L., Lowe, R. and O'Reilly, N. (2017) 'Cervical Rotation Lateral Flexion Test.' *Physiopedia*. Available at www.physio-pedia.com/index.php?title=Cervical_rotation_lateral_flexion_test&oldid=180968

McGee, S.R. (2017) *Evidence-based Physical Diagnosis*. 4th edn. Amsterdam: Elsevier.

McKenzie, R. and May, S. (2006) *The Cervical and Thoracic Spine: Mechanical Diagnosis and Therapy*. 2 Volume Set. 2nd edn. Waikanae, New Zealand: Spinal Publications.

Menzer, H., Gill, G.K. and Paterson, A. (2015) 'Thoracic spine sports-related injuries.' *Current Sports Medicine Reports* 14(1), 34–40. doi:10.1249/JSR.0000000000000117

Newell, N., Pearce, A.P., Spurrier, E., Gibb, I., Webster, C.E., Clasper, J.C. *et al.* (2018) 'Analysis of isolated transverse process fractures sustained during blast related events.' *Journal of Trauma and Acute Care Surgery*, 1. doi:10.1097/ta.0000000000001815

Ombregt, L. (2013) *A System of Orthopaedic Medicine*. London: Churchill Livingstone Elsevier.

Page, B.J., Hubert, Z.T., Rahm, M. and Leahy, M.J. (2018) 'Thoracic spine fractures and dislocations.' *Medscape*. Available at https://emedicine.medscape.com/article/1267029-clinical

Puentedura, E.J. and O'Grady, W.H. (2015) 'Letter to the editor: "Safety of thrust joint manipulation in the thoracic spine: a systematic review."' *Journal of Manual & Manipulative Therapy 23*(4), 174–175. doi:10.1179/2042618615y.0000000018

Rhon, D., Greenlee, T. and Fritz, J. (2018) 'Utilization of manipulative treatment for spine and shoulder conditions between different medical providers in a large military hospital.' *Archives of Physical Medicine and Rehabilitation 99*(1), 72–81. doi:10.1016/J.APMR.2017.06.010

Saker, E., Graham, R.A., Nicholas, R., D'Antoni, A.V., Loukas, M., Oskouian, R.J. *et al.* (2016) 'Ligaments of the costovertebral joints including biomechanics, innervations, and clinical applications: A comprehensive review with application to approaches to the thoracic spine.' *Cureus 8*(11). doi:10.7759/cureus.874

Singh, A., Tetrault, L., Kalsi-Ryan, S., Nouri, A. and Fehlings, M.G. (2014) 'Global prevalence and incidence of traumatic spinal cord injury.' *Clinical Epidemiology 6*, 309. doi:10.2147/CLEP. S68889

Starkey, C. and Brown, S.D. (2010) *Examination of Orthopedic and Athletic Injuries*. Philadelphia, PA: F.A. Davis Co. Available at www.fadavis.com/product/athletic-training-examination-orthopedic-athletic-injuries-starkey-brown-ryan-3

Thornton, C.W. (2018) *The Effects of Thoracic Manipulation in the Treatment of Mechanical Neck Pain: A Meta-analysis*. Fresno, CA: California State University. Available at https://repository. library.fresnostate.edu/bitstream/handle/10211.3/203863/Thornton_csu_6050D_10537. pdf?sequence=1

Watts, E. (2016) 'Thoracolumbar Fracture-Dislocation.' *Orthobullets*. Available at www. orthobullets.com/spine/2024/thoracolumbar-fracture-dislocation

WHO (World Health Organization) (2005) *WHO Guidelines on Basic Training and Safety in Chiropractic*. Geneva: WHO.

Wilke, H.J., Herkommer, A., Werner, K. and Liebsch, C. (2017) 'In vitro analysis of the segmental flexibility of the thoracic spine.' *PLOS One 12*(5), 1–16. doi:10.1371/journal.pone.0177823

CERVICO-THORACIC JUNCTION MANIPULATION TECHNIQUES

Prone cervico-thoracic junction manipulation

- The patient is in the prone position, with their arms over the side of the table.

- The therapist stands in a split-leg stance, with the left leg in front, at the head of the table.

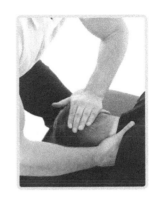

- With your right hand, gently rest the web of your hand over the patient's trapezius, but you do not need to press against the spinous process (SP) of the target segment. Place your left hand against the side of the patient's head just above the ear, ensuring your forearm is parallel with the head of the table.

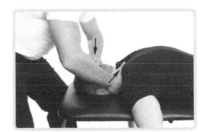

- Ask the patient to inhale and then slowly exhale.

- As the patient starts to exhale, begin to introduce a side-bending force with your right hand through T1 as your left hand simultaneously introduces a rotational force to engage the barrier.

- When the barrier has been engaged, a manipulation is applied through both hands.

Key to note:

- This technique can also be completed by facing the head of the table in an asymmetrical stance and placing your contact hand via your ulnar border into the web of the trapezius, performing the rotation as above.

- Avoid pushing the patient's head onto the table as this becomes uncomfortable.

Side-lying cervico-thoracic junction manipulation, contra-lateral side

- Stand in an asymmetrical stance (outside leg facing forwards), facing the patient.

- Place the pisiform of your right hand over the TP of the target segment, reinforced as shown.

- Ask the patient to breathe in and out.

- On the out breath, engage the barrier by adding oblique inferior pressure, as shown.

- After the barrier is engaged, perform the manipulation in the direction shown.

- This manipulation is performed for the contra-lateral side of the target segment.

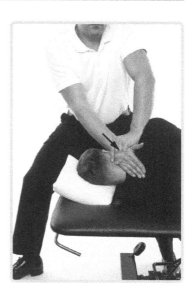

Key to note:

- The barrier can be difficult to feel when first attempting this technique, so avoid using excessive pressure and force.

Seated cervico-thoracic junction manipulation, suboccipital and mastoid contact

- This technique is performed with the patient seated and the therapist standing behind.

- Your right hand circumvents the face of the patient to contact the contra-lateral suboccipital ridge or mastoid process, as shown.

- Your left hand contacts the ipsilateral, lateral SP of T1.

- The contact of your left hand is to stabilise and block the movement of T1.

- Ask the patient to breathe in and out.

- Towards the end of the breath out, engage the barrier by performing rotation of the cervical spine with your right hand while stabilising T1 with your left hand, as shown.

- Perform the manipulation when the barrier is engaged via rotation of the cervical spine.

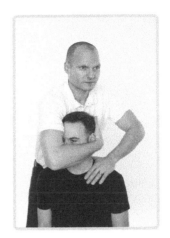

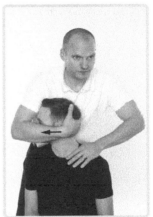

Key to note:

- Thorough screening and testing is needed for the cervical spine due to the rotational aspect.

- Avoid excessive rotation of the cervical spine.

- Avoid excessive pressure of the TP of the T1.

- You may want to place a towel or pillow over your chest to provide comfort for you and the patient.

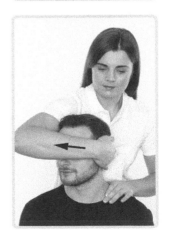

THORACIC SPINE MANIPULATION TECHNIQUES

Supine ipsilateral thoracic manipulation, T2-T12

- You need to have an asymmetrical stance.

- The patient crosses their arms into a 'V' position.

- Slightly rotate the patient away from the side that you are standing on via the superior angle of the scapula, to expose the SPs of the thoracic spine.

- Using your chosen hand position (closed hand, pistol grip or flat hand), contact the segment below your target – that is, T6 to manipulate T5.

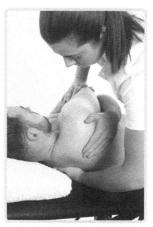

- Your other hand now gently holds the patient's elbows, as you will need to control this to complete the manipulation.

- The patient should now inhale and exhale.

- Halfway through the exhalation breath, roll the patient back towards you and onto your applicator.

- As you roll the patient onto your applicator, compress the patient's elbows via your xiphoid process. The aim is to direct the patient's elbows directly above your applicator.

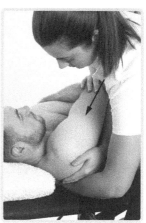

- At the end of the exhalation breath, maximum compression via the elbows should be achieved and the manipulation should be completed.

- The direction of the manipulation is downwards towards your applicator and through the shoulders.

Key to note:

- The 'V' position of the arms allows for greater control and aids force transference during the technique.

- You can assess your target segment by palpating the SPs and gently and slowly rocking the patient on and off your hand.

- A towel can be placed under the crossed arms for people with longer arms or very mobile shoulders.

- A towel can be placed over the patient's elbows to provide a protective cushion for the therapist.

- Maximum compression is achieved via the legs and not your hand.

- The height of the table is very important, requiring enough room to manipulate.

Single supine thoracic manipulation, T2-T12

- You need to have an asymmetrical stance.

- The patient crosses *one* arm into a 'V' position. The other arm is left by their side, as shown.

- Palpate the opposite medial border of the scapula to expose the SPs of the thoracic spine.

- Using your chosen applicator, contact the segment below your target – that is, T6 to manipulate T5.

- Your other hand now gently holds the patient's elbow as you will need to control this to complete the manipulation.

- The patient should now inhale and exhale.

- Halfway through the exhalation breath, roll the patient onto your applicator.

- As you roll the patient onto your applicator, compress the patient's elbows via your xiphoid process. The aim is to direct the patient's elbow directly above your applicator.

- At the end of the exhalation breath, maximum compression via the elbows should be achieved and the manipulation should be completed.

- The direction of the manipulation is downwards towards your applicator and via the shoulder.

Key to note:

- The 'V' position of the arm allows for greater control and aids force transference during the technique.

- You can assess your target segment by palpating the SPs and gently and slowly rocking the patient on and off your hand.

- A towel can be placed under the crossed arms for people with longer arms or very mobile shoulders.

- A towel can be placed over the patient's elbows to provide a protective cushion for the therapist.

- Maximum compression is achieved via the legs and not your hand.

- The height of the table is very important, requiring enough room to manipulate.

Recumbent supine thoracic manipulation, T2-T12

- You need to have an asymmetrical stance.

- The patient crosses their arms into a 'V' position.

- Incline the head of the table to approximately 30°.

- Add a small towel, as shown.

- Slightly rotate the patient away from the side you are standing on via the superior angle of the scapula to expose the SPs of the thoracic spine.

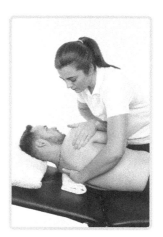

- Using your chosen applicator, contact the segment below your target – that is, T6 to manipulate T5.

- Your other hand now gently holds the patient's elbows as you will need to control this to complete the manipulation.

- The patient should now inhale and exhale.

- Halfway through the exhalation breath, roll the patient back towards you and onto your applicator.

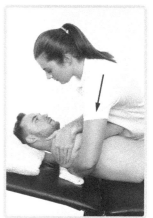

- As you roll the patient onto your applicator, compress the patient's elbows via your xiphoid process. The aim is to direct the patient's elbows directly above your applicator.

- At the end of the exhalation breath, maximum compression via the elbows should be achieved and the manipulation should be completed.

- The direction of the manipulation is downwards towards your applicator and through the shoulders.

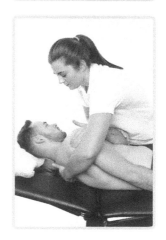

Key to note:

- The 'V' position of the arms allows for greater control and aids force transference during the technique.

- You can also complete this with the patient having a single arm across their chest.

- You can assess your target segment by palpating the SPs and gently and slowly rocking the patient on and off your hand.

- A towel can be placed under the crossed arms for people with longer arms or very mobile shoulders.

- A towel can be placed over the patient's elbows to provide a protective cushion for the therapist.

- Inclining the table can make the technique more comfortable for the patient.

- A small towel under your hand makes it more comfortable as it gives a small, flat surface to lay your hand on.

- Maximum compression is achieved via the legs and not your hand.

- The height of the table is very important, requiring enough room to manipulate.

Rolling supine ipsilateral thoracic manipulation, T2-T12

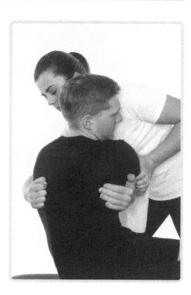

- Start with the patient seated.

- You need to have an asymmetrical stance.

- The patient crosses their arms into a 'V' position.

- Slightly rotate the patient towards you, while holding their elbows.

- From the ipsilateral side, place your chosen applicator on the segment below your target – that is, T6 to manipulate T5.

- Your other hand now gently holds the patient's elbows as you will need to control this to complete the manipulation.

- The patient should now inhale and exhale.

- Halfway through the exhalation breath, roll the patient back towards the midline down towards the table and onto your applicator.

- As your applicator makes contact with the table, compress the patient's elbows via your xiphoid process. The aim is to direct the patient's elbows directly above your applicator.

- At the end of the exhalation breath, maximum compression via the patient's elbows should be achieved and the manipulation should be completed.

- The direction of the manipulation is downwards towards your applicator and through the shoulders.

Key to note:

- This is a dynamic movement and should be applied carefully.

- The benefit of this is to use gravity and momentum to aid you in the manipulation, if needed.

- The 'V' position of the arms allows for greater control and aids force transference during the technique.

- You can also complete this with the patient having a single arm across their chest.

- You can assess your target segment by palpating the SPs and gently and slowly rocking the patient on and off your hand.

- A towel can be placed under the crossed arms for people with longer arms or very mobile shoulders.

- A towel can be placed over the patient's elbows to provide a protective cushion for the therapist.

- Inclining the table can make the technique more comfortable for the patient.

- A small towel under your hand makes it more comfortable as it gives a small, flat surface to lay your hand on.

- Maximum compression is achieved via the legs and not your hand.

- The height of the table is very important, requiring enough room to manipulate.

Reinforced rolling supine ipsilateral thoracic manipulation, T2-T12

- Start with the patient seated.

- You need to have an asymmetrical stance.

- The patient crosses their arms into a 'V' position.

- Slightly rotate the patient towards you, while holding their elbows.

- From the ipsilateral side place your chosen applicator on the segment below your target – that is, T6 to manipulate T5.

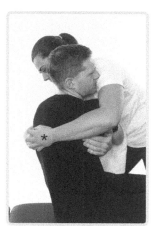

- Your other hand now covers your applicator to support and reinforce.

- The patient should now inhale and exhale.

- Halfway through the exhalation breath, roll the patient back towards the midline down towards the table and onto your applicator.

- As your applicator makes contact with the table, compress the patient's elbows via your xiphoid process. The aim is to direct the patient's elbows directly above your applicator.

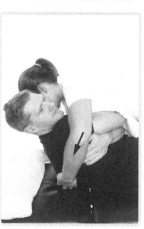

- At the end of the exhalation breath, maximum compression via the patient's elbows should be achieved and the manipulation should be completed.

- The direction of the manipulation is downwards towards your applicator and through the shoulders.

Key to note:

- This is a dynamic movement and should be applied carefully.

- The benefit of this is to use gravity and momentum to aid you in the manipulation, if needed.

- The 'V' position of the arms allows for greater control and aids force transference during the technique.

- You can also complete this with the patient having a single arm across their chest.

- You can assess your target segment by palpating the SPs and gently and slowly rocking the patient on and off your hand.

- A towel can be placed under the crossed arms for people with longer arms or very mobile shoulders.

- A towel can be placed over the patient's elbows to provide a protective cushion for the therapist.

- Inclining the table can make the technique more comfortable for the patient.

- A small towel under your hand makes it more comfortable as it gives a small, flat surface to lay your hand on.

- Maximum compression is achieved via the legs and not your hand.

- The height of the table is very important, requiring enough room to manipulate.

Prone thoracic thrust - 'butterfly', with body drop, T2-T10

- Stand at the side of the table, facing the patient, who is lying in prone position.

- Ensure you have an asymmetrical stance with your lead leg in contact with the table.

- Locate the target segment.

- Your dominant hand should contact the transverse process of the target segment on the ipsilateral side via your pisiform.

- With the other hand, contact the TP of the segment below your target on the contra-lateral side via your pisiform, creating your 'butterfly' wings (i.e., ipsilateral contact on T3 and contra-lateral contact on T4).

- While adding minimal contact on the patient, ask them to inhale.

- Ask the patient to inhale and exhale. As the patient exhales, begin to move your bodyweight over the target segment. Imagine you are aiming to place your xiphoid process over the SP.

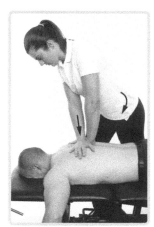

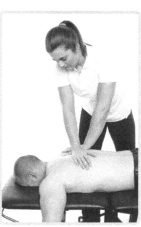

- As you follow the exhalation breath, add equal bilateral compression through both arms, which are at almost full extension, and external rotation of both your shoulders to gather any skin slack.

- As the patient reaches full exhalation, apply your manipulation while rotating your hips through towards the table, as shown.

Key to note:

- For patient comfort you may want to place a small towel under each shoulder.

- Breathing is key. Allow the patient to inhale while you apply minimal compression, and as they exhale, gradually increase compression by moving your bodyweight forwards, over the target segment.

- At the full end point of exhalation, ensuring there is minimal air left in the lungs, apply your manipulation.

- This is a great technique to use when the patient is much bigger than you and you may need a little extra momentum to achieve the manipulation.

Prone thoracic spear technique with body drop, T2-T12

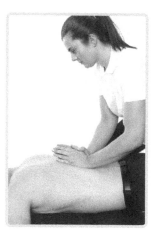

- It can be applied with the therapist either at the side or at the head of the table.

- The technique can be applied inferior-superior (IS) and superior-inferior (SI) from the top of the table (mostly done as shown).

- You should have an asymmetrical stance.

- Your applicator (bilateral aspect of pisiform) should contact the TP of the target with both arms at almost full extension.

- Aim to have your xiphoid process over the target segment as far as possible.

- Ask the patient to inhale and exhale.

- Halfway through the exhalation breath, begin to engage the barrier by adding a downward and oblique compression.

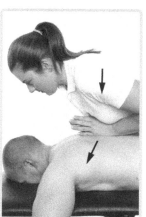

- At the end of the exhalation breath, the barrier should be engaged and you should manipulate the target joint by dropping your upper body through your hands, as shown.

Key to note:

- Use your legs in order to add the necessary compression to engage the barrier.

- Remember to work with the patient's breathing (this is vitally important, to decrease intrathecal pressure).

- Add the full downward compression at the very end of exhalation.

Prone thoracic spear technique body drop with extension, T2-T12

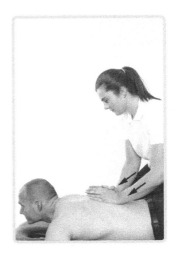

- It can be applied with the therapist either at the side or head of the table.

- The technique can be applied IS or SI from the top of the table (mostly done as shown).

- You should have an asymmetrical stance.

- Your applicator (bilateral aspect of pisiform) should contact the TP of the target with both arms at almost full extension.

- Aim to have your xiphoid process over the target segment as far as possible.

- The patient is then asked to move their cervical and thoracic spine into extension.

- Ask the patient to inhale and exhale.

- Halfway through the exhalation breath, begin to engage the barrier by adding a downward and oblique compression.

- At the end of the exhalation breath, the barrier should be engaged and you should manipulate the target joint by dropping your upper body through your hands, as shown.

Key to note:

- Use your legs in order to add the necessary compression to engage the barrier.

- Stop the patient moving into extension when you feel your target move towards you.

- You do not need a lot of extension; it's less than you think.

- Remember to work with the patient's breathing (this is vitally important, to decrease intrathecal pressure).

- Add the full downward compression at the very end of exhalation.

Single hand thoracic manipulation, T2-T12

- It can be applied with the therapist either at the side or head of the table.

- The technique can be applied IS or SI from the top of the table (mostly done as shown).

- You should have an asymmetrical stance.

- Your hand should contact over the SP, slightly cupping it in your thenar eminence (not directly on it as this can be uncomfortable), at almost full extension.

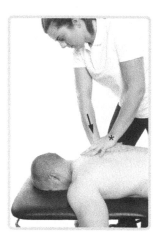

- Your other hand stabilises and supports your contact hand, as shown.

- Aim to have your xiphoid process over the target segment as far as possible.

- Ask the patient to inhale and exhale.

- Halfway through the exhalation breath, begin to engage the barrier by adding a downward and oblique compression.

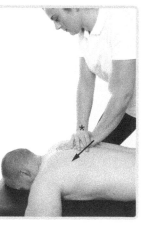

- At the end of the exhalation breath, the barrier should be engaged and you should manipulate the target joint by dropping your upper body through your hands, as shown.

Key to note:

- Beware – the higher you apply this technique to the thoracic spine, the more likely you are to begin to push the patient's throat towards the face hole, so confirm comfort throughout.

- You have two different hand positions for this technique, as shown.

- Use your legs in order to add the necessary compression to engage the barrier.

- Stop the patient moving into extension when you feel your target move towards you.

- Remember to work with the patient's breathing (this is vitally important, to decrease intrathecal pressure).

- Add the full downward compression at the very end of exhalation.

Double hand thoracic manipulation, T2-T12

- It can be applied with the therapist either at the side or head of the table.

- The technique can be applied IS or SI from the top of the table (mostly done as shown).

- You should have an asymmetrical stance.

- Your hand should contact over the TPs of the target segment, as shown, with your elbows at almost full extension.

- Aim to have your xiphoid process over the target segment as far as possible.

- Ask the patient to inhale and exhale.

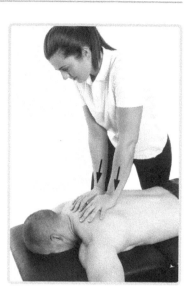

- Halfway through the exhalation breath, begin to engage the barrier by adding a downward and oblique compression.

- At the end of the exhalation phase, the barrier should be engaged and you should manipulate the target joint by dropping your upper body through your hands, as shown.

Key to note:

- Beware – the higher you apply this technique to the thoracic spine, the more likely you are to begin to push the patient's throat towards the face hole, so confirm comfort throughout.

- Use your legs in order to add the necessary compression to engage the barrier.

- Stop the patient moving into extension when you feel your target move towards you.

- Remember to work with the patient's breathing (this is vitally important, to decrease intrathecal pressure).

- Add the full downward compression at the very end of exhalation.

Standing ipsilateral thoracic manipulation, T2-T12

- The patient stands with their back to the wall, as shown.

- You need to have an asymmetrical stance.

- The patient crosses their arms into a 'V' position.

- Slightly rotate the patient away you from on the side you are standing on, via their elbows, to expose the SPs of the thoracic spine.

- Using your chosen applicator, contact the segment below your target – that is, T6 to manipulate T5 from the ipsilateral side.

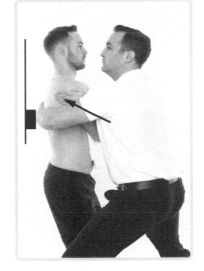

- Your other hand now gently holds the patient's elbows as you will need to control this to complete the manipulation.

- The patient should now inhale and exhale.

- Halfway through the exhalation phase, roll the patient back towards you and onto your applicator.

- As you roll the patient onto your applicator, compress the patient's elbows via your xiphoid process. The aim is to direct the patient's elbows directly above your applicator.

- At the end of the exhalation phase, maximum compression via the elbows should be achieved and the manipulation should be completed.

- The direction of the manipulation is towards your applicator and through the shoulders.

Key to note:

- Ideally place a pad on the wall to protect your hand.

- Choose the wall carefully – a false wall is not the best choice for this technique.

- This is an excellent technique if you are limited for space or if the patient is too acute to lie down.

- You can apply this technique with a patient's single arm across their chest.

- You can assess your target segment by palpating the SPs and gently and slowly rocking the patient on and off your hand.

- A towel can be placed under the crossed arms for people with longer arms or very mobile shoulders.

- A towel can be placed over the patient's elbows to provide a protective cushion for the therapist.

- Maximum compression is achieved via the legs and not your hand.

6

SHOULDER AND RIB CAGE

Introduction

The concept of regional interdependence suggests that musculoskeletal disorders may be managed better with a regional examination and treatment approach in addition to localised treatment (Strunce *et al.* 2009; Wassinger *et al.* 2016). This approach is frequently employed by manual therapists addressing musculoskeletal complaints of the shoulder girdles and rib cage as these areas tend to have great sympathy, with pain in one area likely to affect the other. This is commonly the case with individuals complaining of shoulder pain as they often have minimised thoracic mobility compared with those who do not present symptoms (Haik, Alburquerque-Sendín and Camargo 2017).

Studies have shown that the addition of manipulative therapy to the medical care of patients reporting pain and dysfunction of the shoulder and rib areas significantly improves short- and long-term recovery rates and lowers the severity of symptoms for these subjects (Strunce *et al.* 2009; Wassinger *et al.* 2016). High-velocity, low-amplitude thrust (HVLAT) manipulation techniques are commonly employed in the treatment of shoulder and thoracic dysfunction by chiropractors and other therapists, with positive results being reported by patients (Gibbons and Tehan 2006). However, a recent review of thrust manipulation for managing shoulder pain expressed the need for more high-quality studies to further explore these manipulation techniques (Minkalis *et al.* 2017).

An understanding of the biomechanics of the rib cage is key to all forms of treatment for multiple conditions, and equally important is an appreciation of the basic anatomy of the ribs (Lee 2015; Liebsch *et al.* 2017). The thoracic skeleton is an irregularly shaped osteocartilaginous cylinder consisting of the flat sternum anteroventrally, 12 pairs of ribs and their associated costal cartilages as well as 12 thoracic vertebrae and intervening vertebral discs that stabilise the thoracic spine (Standring 2016; Yoganandan and Pintar 1998). The thoracic cage protects the heart, lungs and other vital organs that are located within the thoracic cavity, and it serves as an attachment site for various muscles (OpenStax 2018; Sham *et al.* 2005; Yoganandan and Pintar 1998). The ribs are classified into two main categories – namely, typical and atypical (Graeber and Nazim 2007). Typical ribs connect with the sternum anteriorly via costal cartilages (through a cup) and the spinal column posteriorly, forming a thoracic ring consisting of 13 joints (Lee 2015). The typical ribs have characteristic features such as a head, neck, tubercle, articular facet, shaft and a bottom notch housing the neurovascular bundle (intercostal nerve, an artery and a vein).

Atypical ribs, on the other hand, consist of the first two pairs (ribs 1 and 2) that are joined to the cylinder and floating ribs (ribs 11 and 12). The first rib is flat, short, sharply curved and has a single facet on the head while rib 2 is somewhat larger and more developed. The floating ribs also have one facet on the head and lack a tubercle, with their ends tapering to rudimentary cartilages (Graeber and Nazim 2007).

In this chapter, HVLAT manipulation of the shoulder and rib region is explored and special attention directed to outlining the various joints and their ranges of motion. Special diagnostic tests, common injuries to the shoulder and rib cage and red flags for manipulation are also outlined. Therapists should always endeavour to use sound judgement and best practices to ensure patient safety and the best outcomes from manipulative therapies.

Joints

The shoulder girdle consists of four bones (i.e., scapula, humerus, sternum, clavicle), and the intricate articulation of three of these at the shoulder joint forms one of the most complex joints of the human body (Garbis 2017). The shoulder is also the point of attachment of the upper appendage to the axial skeleton. Much of the stability of the shoulder joint is due to the rotator cuff muscles (Garbis 2017).

The ribs allow for mobility during respiration due to the costal cartilages, as well as articulation with the sternum and vertebral bones at either end of the rib (Yoganandan and Pintar 1998). In addition to accommodating respiratory mobility, ribs 1 through 7 rotate posteriorly and anteriorly, in full inhalation and full exhalation respectively (Lee 2015). The function and mobility of the different joints of the shoulder and rib cage can be viewed in Table 6.1.

Table 6.1. Joints of the shoulder and rib cage

Joint name	Description	Function
Glenohumeral joint	• Connects the upper limb to the axis of the body • A highly mobile ball-and-socket joint involving articulation of the head of the humerus with the lateral scapula • Joint surfaces are mismatched and asymmetrical • Has several static and dynamic restraints to the range of motion including muscles (rotator cuff and periscapular), the joint capsule, glenoid labrum, articular surfaces and ligaments (coracohumeral and glenohumeral)	• Allows an extensive amount of mobility to position the arm in space • Allows for various upper extremity motions including rotation (circular, lateral and medial), abduction, adduction, flexion and extension
Acromioclavicular joint	• The lateral end of the clavicle articulates with the medial end of the acromion to form this synovial joint • The articular ends of both bones are covered with fibrocartilage • The acromioclavicular ligament provides anterior and posterior stability while coracoclavicular ligaments (trapezoid and conoid) provide vertical stabilisation • A meniscoid articular disc covers the superior section of the joint	• Stabilises the shoulder and contributes to the arm's movement • Plays an intermediary role in transmission of forces between the clavicle and acromion
Sternoclavicular joint	• This is a synovial joint connecting the sternum's superior portion and the clavicle's medial aspect • This articulation is the only bony connection between the axial skeleton and the upper limb, and it is considered a saddle joint as well as a ball-and-socket joint • Ligamentous restraints of the joint include the posterior sternoclavicular ligament and the costoclavicular ligament that limits superior migration of the clavicle • An articular disc is located between the medial end of the clavicle and the sternum	• Allows free movement of the clavicle in almost all anatomical planes • Its anatomy allows for forward thrust of the shoulder
Costovertebral joint	• Yet another synovial joint connecting the ribs with the costal facets of their respective vertebral bodies • These joints encompass a fibrous capsule, as well as the radiate and interarticular ligaments	• Stabilises the thoracic spine in the three main anatomical planes • Serves to support spinal movement • Allows synchronisation of rib functioning during pulmonary ventilation

Costochondral joint	• This is the joint that attaches the ribs to the costal cartilages • Composed of hyaline cartilage	• Stabilises the rib cage
Costotransverse joint	• These are synovial joints formed between the tubercle of the rib and the transverse process of the vertebra of the same level • Supported by the superior costotransverse ligament, costotransverse ligament and lateral costotransverse ligament • Not present in T11 and T12 as the ribs at this level do not articulate with transverse processes	• Facilitates concomitant rib motion during breathing

Sources: Garbis (2017); Magee (2014); Sham et al. (2005)

Range of motion

The glenohumeral joint of the shoulder is the most moveable articulation in humans as it allows for a great variety of movements including rotation (both internal and external), forward flexion, extension, abduction and adduction (Werner *et al.* 2014) (see Table 6.2). However, the high mobility of the shoulder joint also makes it the most unstable joint (Garbis 2017).

Table 6.2. Typical ranges of motion in the shoulder

Motion type	Range of motion
Forward flexion	180°
Extension	45–60°
Abduction	150°
Internal rotation	70–90°
External rotation	90°

Source: Adapted from Moses (2007)

The rib cage has a stabilising effect on the thoracic spine, and this results in a more limited range of motion (Liebsch *et al.* 2017; Sham *et al.* 2005). In a recent study, the range of motion of the thoracic spine in its intact condition with the rib cage attached showed median values of 10.5° of flexion/extension, 14.9° of lateral bending and 20.4° of axial rotation (Liebsch *et al.* 2017). In the same study it was demonstrated that removal of the rib components had the expected effect of an increase in the range of motion of the thoracic spine (Liebsch *et al.* 2017).

Common injuries

Injuries to the shoulder and rib cage often occur as a result of motor vehicle accidents, injuries from sporting activities, or other forms of trauma. These traumatic injuries may result in soft tissue damage and fracturing of bones, resulting in pain and reduced mobility. The shoulder is prone to injury because it lacks the stability to allow its wide range of motion (Garbis 2017; Kahn and Xu 2017). It is little surprise that shoulder injuries are commonly observed among the general populace and more so in athletes who frequently make complex motions with their upper extremities in competitive sport. The rib cage, on the other hand, is not so moveable but it is often indicated in injury due to the various aforementioned factors. Table 6.3 summarises the common injuries of both these body areas.

Table 6.3. Common injuries of the shoulder and rib cage

Common injuries	Incidence	Characteristics
Glenohumeral dislocation	• 23.9 per 100,000 person-years (USA) • 28.02 per 100,000 person-years (UK)	• Results from disarticulation of the contact between the humerus head and the glenoid fossa • It is estimated that anterior dislocations account for 96% of all shoulder dislocations, with posterior dislocations making up the difference
Clavicle fracture	• 30–60 cases per 100,000 population globally • 3.3 per 10,000 person-years (UK)	• This is a common acute injury usually associated with falls on the lateral shoulder • Shows a male dominance pattern of approximately 70%
Acromioclavicular sprain	• 1.8 per 10,000 person-years (USA)	• Common in physically active people including athletes • Results from direct trauma to the acromion with an adducted humerus • More frequent in males compared with females, with a 5:1 ratio, and a greater frequency of occurrence in 20- to 30-year-olds

Proximal humerus fracture	• 31 per 100,000 person-years (UK) • 82 per 100,000 person-years (USA)	• Infrequent and characterised with poor prognosis • Frequently results from falling onto an extended arm • Greater incidence in the elderly population
Rib fracture	• 3.8 per 10,000 person-years (UK) • 6.3 per 10,000 person-years (USA)	• Commonly an effect of trauma to the chest • Also attributed to coughing or forceful muscular contraction of the body's axis and upper extremity • Ribs 7 and 10 are the most commonly affected • Characterised by high-intensity local pain at the fracture site, and pain in respiratory motions

Sources: *Chillemi et al. (2013); Curtis et al. (2016); Eastell et al. (2001); Kahn and Xu (2017); Kihlström et al. (2017); Launonen et al. (2015); Shah et al. (2017); Sirin, Aydin and Mert Topkar (2018); van der Velde et al. (2016); Zacchilli and Owens (2010)*

Red flags

Red flags are signs and symptoms that point to serious underlying pathology in patients with chronic pain (Monga and Funk 2017). When red flags (see Table 6.4) have been diagnosed in a patient, the therapist should exercise sound clinical reasoning and caution, to minimise the patient's risk of adverse effects following manipulation.

Table 6.4. Red flags for serious pathology in the shoulder and rib cage

Condition	Signs and symptoms
Acute rotator cuff tear	• Pain following trauma • Acute disabling pain in the shoulder, sensory deficits • Considerable muscle weakness • A positive drop arm test
Neurological lesion	• Unexplained muscular wasting • Neurological insufficiency (e.g., sensory or motor) • Importunate headaches
Radiculopathy	• Severe radiating pain • Tingling sensation in shoulder

Condition	Signs and symptoms
Dropped head syndrome	• Intense weakness of neck extensor muscle • Flexor muscle sparing • Chin-on-chest deformity • Neck muscle inflexibility • Shoulder weakness
Unreduced dislocation	• Severe trauma • Epilepsy • Electric shock • Rotation loss and deformity
Myocardial infarction	• Chest pain or discomfort • Thoracic tension • Shortness of breath, perspiring, sallowness, shaking, faintness and nausea
Pericarditis	• Sharp thoracic pain towards the medial or left region • Pain associated with normal physiologic activities such as breathing (especially deep inspiration), swallowing and coughing • Relief when leaning forward and sitting upright • Shortness of breath, exhaustion, queasiness, heart palpitations
Pneumothorax	• Intense thoracic pain with pulmonary respiration or rib cage expansion • Hasty breathing • Low blood pressure, dyspnoea or hypoxia • Faint or absent breath sounds
Pneumonia	• Penetrating chest pain associated with breathing or coughing • Fever, tremors, headache, perspiring, exhaustion or nausea • Expectoration
Fracture	• >70 years of age • Recent history of major trauma • Protracted corticosteroids use • History of osteoporosis
Tumour	• History of cancer (e.g., breast carcinoma and lung carcinoma) • Suspected malignancy • Unexplained deformity, mass or swelling

Infection, septic arthritis	• Inflammation
	• Malaise and exhaustion
	• Loss of appetite, fever, chills
	• Sudden weight loss
	• Recent history of bacterial infection
	• Intense and/or persistent shoulder complaints

Sources: Dutton (2016); Kahn and Xu (2017); Magee (2014); Mitchell et al. (2005); Shanley et al. (2015)

Special tests

This section summarises some of the most commonly used tests to assess for instability of the shoulder and rib cage (see Table 6.5). Therapists are encouraged to familiarise themselves with these tests to properly apply them and correctly interpret the results for the benefit of the patient.

This table is not an exhaustive list of special tests but gives you, the therapist, a guide for this area. If you are unsure of the interpretation of any test that you complete with your patient, we advise that you refer to the most appropriate medical professional for further investigations.

Table 6.5. Special tests for shoulder and rib cage dysfunction

Test	Procedure	Positive sign	Interpretation
Hawkins–Kennedy test Specificity: 0.25 Sensitivity: 0.69	The therapist flexes the patient's shoulder in front of the body to 90°. The therapist then internally rotates the shoulder at the glenohumeral joint	• Pain in the deltoid area • Pain radiating down the arm	✓ Internal impingement ✓ Tendinitis and bursitis
Drop arm test Specificity: 0.88 Sensitivity: 0.35	The therapist passively abducts the patient's arm to 160°. The patient is then instructed to slowly lower the arm to the waist	• Inability to control the manoeuvre as far as the side	✓ Supraspinatus or rotator cuff tear
Apprehension test Specificity: 0.71 Sensitivity: 0.98	The patient assumes a supine or sitting position. The therapist passively moves the shoulder into external rotation while the arm is held at 90° of abduction and the elbow flexed to a right angle	• A sensation of apprehension accompanied by a feeling that the shoulder may dislocate	✓ Glenohumeral instability ✓ Tear of the anterior labrum

Test	Procedure	Positive sign	Interpretation
Jobe's empty can test Specificity: 0.78 Sensitivity: 0.97	The therapist performs this test with the patient's shoulders in 90° of abduction, 30° forward flexion and internal rotation such that the thumb points to the floor The test may be performed both passively and against active resistance	• Weakness in comparison with the contra-lateral limb • Inability to maintain the test position passively	✓ Supraspinatus tear or rotator cuff impingement
Anterior-posterior rib compression test	The patient assumes a sitting or standing position. The therapist stands to the side of the patient with their hands on the anterior and posterior aspects of the rib cage, applies pressure with both hands and then releases the pressure	• Rib shaft prominence in midaxillary line • A feeling of pain or point tenderness with compression • Respiratory restrictions	✓ Potential rib fracture, contusion or costochondral separation
Chest expansion test	The patient may be seated or standing. The therapist locates their thumbs close to the patient's 10th ribs with the fingers parallel to the lateral rib cage and barely grasping the lower hemithorax on both sides of the axilla. With gentle pressure, the therapist slides their hands in the medial direction, elevating a loose skin fold between the thumbs, and asks the patient to take a deep breath and expire fully The therapist then moves to stand in front of the patient while placing their thumbs to each costal margin laterally. With their hands now along the lateral rib cage, the therapist slides them medially to again elevate a loose skin fold between the thumbs. The patient repeats the deep inspiration and expiration. The therapist must note the space between the thumbs in both posterior and anterior aspects while feeling for the symmetry of motion of the hemithorax	• Asymmetrical chest expansion • Less expansion on the abnormal side • Slow expansion compared with the normal side	✓ Unilateral reduction or a prolonging of chest expansion is indicative of pathology including but not limited to lobar pneumonia, pleural effusion and unilateral bronchial obstruction ✓ Bilateral reduction in chest expansion is suggestive of chronic obstructive pulmonary disease or asthma

Rib cage respiratory test	Ribs 1–10: With the patient assuming a supine posture, the therapist palpates over the ribs anteriorly, giving special attention to the intercostal spaces. The patient then takes a deep breath with full expiration. The therapist assesses the respiratory excursion for the superior and inferior ribs	• Rib motion stops during either inhalation or exhalation	✓ Rib dysfunction
	Ribs 11 and 12: The patient assumes a prone position and the therapist places their hand symmetrically over the 11th and 12th ribs posteriorly. The patient takes another deep breath with full expiration. The therapist proceeds to palpate the motion while assessing the respiratory excursion		

Sources: Flynn (1996); Garbis (2017); Hattam and Smeatham (2010); Kahn and Xu (2017); Magee (2014); Monga and Funk (2017); Tovin and Greenfield (2001)

The shoulder girdle is both highly mobile and unstable, which makes it particularly prone to injury. This is especially true of athletes participating in competitive sports who often present with injuries of the shoulder region. For effective treatment, it is necessary for therapists to carefully examine any potential injuries without exacerbating the condition. While the rib cage may not be as mobile as the shoulder region, it is nonetheless a delicate structure. Injuries to the thoracic cage may have far-reaching impacts as this stabilises the body's axis and protects the vital organs. A thorough understanding of regional anatomy is thus recommended in order to apply the most appropriate treatment modality or refer for further assessment.

References

Chillemi, C., Francheschini, V., Dei Guidici, L., Alibardi, A., Salate Santone, F., Ramos Alday, L.J. *et al.* (2013) 'Epidemiology of isolated acromioclavicular joint dislocation.' *Emergency Medicine International*, 171609. doi:10.1155/2013/171609

Curtis, E.M., van der Velde, R., Moon, R.J., van der Bergh, J.P., Geusens, P., de Vries, F. *et al.* (2016) 'Epidemiology of fractures in the United Kingdom 1988-2012: Variation with age, sex, geography, ethnicity and socioeconomic status.' *Bone 87*, 19–26. doi:10.1016/j.bone.2016.03.006

Dutton, M. (2016) *Dutton's Orthopaedic Examination, Evaluation, and Intervention.* New York: McGraw-Hill Education.

Eastell, R., Reid, D.M., Compston, J., Cooper, C., Fogelman, I., Francis, R.M. *et al.* (2001) 'Secondary prevention of osteoporosis: When should a non-vertebral fracture be a trigger for action?' *QJM: Monthly Journal of the Association of Physicians* 94(11), 575–597. doi:10.1093/qjmed/94.11.575

Flynn, T.W. (1996) *The Thoracic Spine and Rib Cage: Musculoskeletal Evaluation and Treatment.* Oxford: Butterworth-Heinemann. Available at https://books.google.co.zw/books/about/The_Thoracic_Spine_and_Rib_Cage.html?id=_7xsAAAAMAAJ&redir_esc=y

Garbis, N.G. (2017) 'Surgical Approaches to the Shoulder.' In G. Huri and N.K. Paschos (eds) *The Shoulder.* Cham: Springer International Publishing (Orthopaedic Study Guide Series). doi:10.1007/978-3-319-51979-1

Gibbons, P. and Tehan, P. (2006) *Manipulation of the Spine, Thorax and Pelvis: An Osteopathic Perspective.* 2nd edn. Philadelphia, PA: Churchill Livingstone Elsevier.

Graeber, G.M. and Nazim, M. (2007) 'The anatomy of the ribs and the sternum and their relationship to chest wall structure and function.' *Thoracic Surgery Clinics* 17(4), 473–489. doi:10.1016/j.thorsurg.2006.12.010

Haik, M.N., Alburquerque-Sendín, F. and Camargo, P.R. (2017) 'Short-term effects of thoracic spine manipulation on shoulder impingement syndrome: A randomized controlled trial.' *Archives of Physical Medicine and Rehabilitation* 98(8), 1594–1605. doi:10.1016/j.apmr.2017.02.003

Hattam, P. and Smeatham, A. (2010) *Special Tests in Musculoskeletal Examination: An Evidence-based Guide for Clinicians.* Philadelphia, PA: Churchill Livingstone Elsevier.

Kahn, S.B. and Xu, R.Y. (2017) *Musculoskeletal Sports and Spine Disorders: A Comprehensive Guide.* Cham, Switzerland: Springer. doi:10.1007/978-3-319-50512-1

Kihlström, C., Möller, M., Lönn, K. and Wolf, O. (2017) 'Clavicle fractures: Epidemiology, classification and treatment of 2 422 fractures in the Swedish Fracture Register: An observational study.' *BMC Musculoskeletal Disorders* 18(1), 82. doi:10.1186/s12891-017-1444-1

Launonen, A.P., Lepola, V., Saranko, A., Flinkkilä, T., Laitinen, M. and Mattila, V.M. (2015) 'Epidemiology of proximal humerus fractures.' *Archives of Osteoporosis* 10(1), 1–5. doi:10.1007/s11657-015-0209-4

Lee, D.G. (2015) 'Biomechanics of the thorax – Research evidence and clinical expertise.' *Journal of Manual & Manipulative Therapy* 23(3), 128–138. doi:10.1179/2042618615Y.0000000008

Liebsch, C., Graf, N., Appelt, K. and Wilke, H.-J. (2017) 'The rib cage stabilizes the human thoracic spine: An in vitro study using stepwise reduction of rib cage structures.' *PLOS One* 12(6), e0178733. doi:10.1371/journal.pone.0178733

Magee, D.J. (2014) *Orthopedic Physical Assessment.* 6th edn. St Louis, MO: Saunders.

Minkalis, A.L., Vining, R.D., Long, C.R., Hawk, C. and de Luca, K. (2017) 'A systematic review of thrust manipulation for non-surgical shoulder conditions.' *Chiropractic & Manual Therapies* 25(1), 1. doi:10.1186/s12998-016-0133-8

Mitchell, C., Adebajo, A., Hay, E. and Carr, A. (2005) 'Shoulder pain: Diagnosis and management in primary care.' *British Medical Journal* 331(7525), 1124–1128. doi:10.1136/bmj.331.7525.1124

Monga, P. and Funk, L. (eds) (2017) *Diagnostic Clusters in Shoulder Conditions.* Cham, Switzerland: Springer International Publishing. doi:10.1007/978-3-319-57334-2

Moses, S. (2007) 'Shoulder Range of Motion, Family Practice Notebook.' Available at https://fpnotebook.com/Ortho/Exam/ShldrRngOfMtn.htm

OpenStax (2018) *Anatomy and Physiology.* OpenStax CNX. Available at http://cnx.org/contents/14fb4ad7-39a1-4eee-ab6e-3ef2482e3e22@12.8

Shah, A., Judge, A., Delmestri, A., Edwards, K., Arden, N.K., Prieto-Alhambra, D. *et al.* (2017) 'Incidence of shoulder dislocations in the UK, 1995–2015: A population-based cohort study.' *British Medical Journal Open* 7(11), e016112. doi:10.1136/bmjopen-2017-016112

Sham, M.L., Zander, T., Rohlmann, A. and Bergmann, G. (2005) 'Effects of the rib cage on thoracic spine flexibility.' *Biomedizinische Technik* 50(11), 361–365. doi:10.1515/BMT.2005.051

Shanley, E., Kissenberth, M.J., Thigpen, C.A., Bailey, L.B., Hawkins, R.J., Michener, L.A. *et al.* (2015) 'Preseason shoulder range of motion screening as a predictor of injury among youth and adolescent baseball pitchers.' *Journal of Shoulder and Elbow Surgery 24*(7), 1005–1013. doi:10.1016/j.jse.2015.03.012

Sirin, E., Aydin, N. and Mert Topkar, O. (2018) 'Acromioclavicular joint injuries: Diagnosis, classification and ligamentoplasty procedures.' *EFORT Open Reviews 3*(7), 426–433. doi:10.1302/2058-5241.3.170027

Standring, S. (ed.) (2016) *Gray's Anatomy: The Anatomical Basis of Clinical Practice.* 41st edn. New York: Elsevier. Available at www.elsevier.com/books/grays-anatomy/standring/978-0-7020-5230-9

Strunce, J.B., Walker, M.J., Boyles, R.E. and Young, B.A. (2009) 'The immediate effects of thoracic spine and rib manipulation on subjects with primary complaints of shoulder pain.' *Journal of Manual & Manipulative Therapy 17*(4), 230–236. doi:10.1179/106698109791352102

Tovin, B.J. and Greenfield, B.H. (2001) *Evaluation and Treatment of the Shoulder: An Integration of the Guide to Physical Therapist Practice.* Philadelphia, PA: F.A. Davis Company.

van der Velde, R.Y., Wyers, C.E., Curtis, E.M., Geusens, P.M., van den Burgh, J.P.W., de Vries, F. *et al.* (2016) 'Secular trends in fracture incidence in the UK between 1990 and 2012.' *Osteoporosis International 27*(11), 3197–3206. doi:10.1007/s00198-016-3650-3

Wassinger, C.A., Rich, D., Cameron, N., Clark, S., Davenport, S., Lingelbach, M. *et al.* (2016) 'Cervical and thoracic manipulations: Acute effects upon pain pressure threshold and self-reported pain in experimentally induced shoulder pain.' *Manual Therapy 21*, 227–232. doi:10.1016/j.math.2015.08.009

Werner, B.C., Holzgrefe, R.E., Griffin, J.W., Lyons, M.L., Cosgrove, C.T., Hart, J.M. *et al.* (2014) 'Validation of an innovative method of shoulder range-of-motion measurement using a smartphone clinometer application.' *Journal of Shoulder and Elbow Surgery 23*(11), e275–e282. doi:10.1016/j.jse.2014.02.030

Yoganandan, N. and Pintar, F.A. (1998) 'Biomechanics of human thoracic ribs.' *Journal of Biomechanical Engineering 120*(February), 100–104. doi:10.1115/1.2834288

Zacchilli, M.A. and Owens, B.D. (2010) 'Epidemiology of shoulder dislocations presenting to emergency departments in the United States.' *Journal of Bone and Joint Surgery – Series A 92*(3), 542–549. doi:10.2106/JBJS.I.00450

SHOULDER MANIPULATION TECHNIQUES

Seated acromioclavicular (AC) joint (muscle energy technique and HVLA thrust technique)

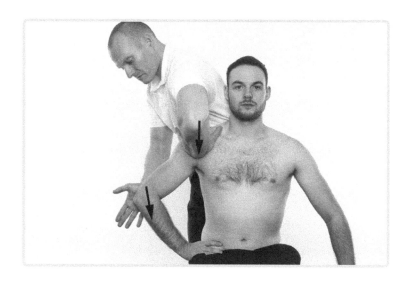

- This technique is applicable for the AC joint with a muscle energy technique using active resisted movement or as a HVLA thrust manipulation.

- The patient is in a seated position with their hand on their hip to stabilise and reinforce, with the therapist standing behind them on the affected side.

- Position yourself against the patient's scapula to stop them leaning backwards, and contact over the AC joint with one hand and the posterior aspect of the patient's elbow with the other.

- Muscle energy technique: stabilise the AC and then push the patient's elbow forwards as the patient actively pushes their elbow back against the resistance, creating a passive cavitation.

- HVLA: stabilise the AC and then push the elbow forwards as the patient actively pushes their elbow back against the resistance; then apply a thrust anteriorly.

Seated acromioclavicular (AC) joint (muscle energy technique and HVLA thrust technique)

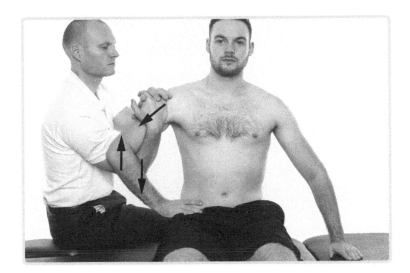

- This technique is applicable for the AC joint with a muscle energy technique using active resisted movement or as a HVLA thrust manipulation.

- The patient is in a seated position with their hand on their hip to stabilise and reinforce, with the therapist standing on the affected side.

- From posterior to anterior you should contact the patient's anterior deltoid, as shown.

- Interlock your hands over the glenohumeral joint and apply light compression to stabilise contacts over the AC joint; your outside arm will be in contact with the posterior aspect of the patient's elbow.

- Ask the patient to lean away from you to gain traction of the glenohumeral joint.

- Muscle energy technique: stabilise the AC and then push the elbow forwards as the patient actively pushes their elbow back against the resistance, creating a passive cavitation.

- HVLA: stabilise the AC and then push the elbow forwards as the patient actively pushes their elbow back against the resistance; then apply a thrust anteriorly.

Seated superior to inferior glenohumeral (GH) and acromioclavicular (AC) joint HVLA

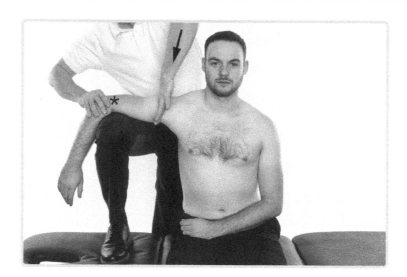

- The patient is in a seated position with the arm of the affected side positioned over the therapist's leg, the therapist standing behind them on the affected side.

- With the patient's arm stabilised over your leg, contact the patient's elbow, and reinforce to reduce movement.

- Your contact hand is slightly inferior to the AC joint, with the elbow high to ensure the line of drive is slightly oblique.

- Take up the skin slack and gain pre-tension by applying a gentle movement from superior to inferior.

- Once pre-tension has been taken up and the restricted barrier reached, the patient should inhale, and then on exhalation apply an HVLA in an oblique inferior direction.

Seated superior to inferior glenohumeral (GH) and acromioclavicular (AC) joint HVLA in flexion

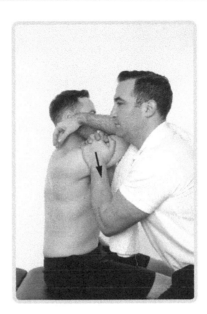

- The patient is in a seated position with the arm of the affected side raised to just above 90°, flexed with the elbow bent; the patient's hand should not rest on their shoulder.

- Stand in front of them on the affected side, in a lunge stance.

- The patient's elbow is stabilised over your shoulder.

- Your contact hands are slightly inferior to the AC joint.

- The patient's elbow is being used as a fulcrum/pivot for the technique.

- Take up the skin slack and gain pre-tension by applying a gentle movement from superior to inferior.

- Once pre-tension has been taken up and the restricted barrier reached, the patient should inhale, and then on exhalation apply an HVLA in an oblique inferior direction.

Seated superior to inferior glenohumeral (GH) and acromioclavicular (AC) joint HVLA in flexion with straight arm

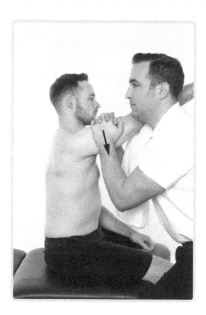

- The patient is in a seated position with the arm of the affected side raised to just above 90°; the patient's arm is positioned straight out, with their elbow supported and in contact with the therapist's shoulder.

- Stand in front of them on the affected side, in a lunge stance.

- Your contact hands are slightly inferior to the AC joint.

- The patient's elbow is being used as a fulcrum/pivot for the technique.

- Take up the skin slack and gain pre-tension by applying a gentle movement from superior to inferior.

- Once pre-tension has been taken up and the restricted barrier reached, the patient should inhale, and then on exhalation apply an HVLA in an oblique inferior direction.

Seated superior to inferior glenohumeral (GH) and acromioclavicular (AC) joint HVLA in abduction with straight arm

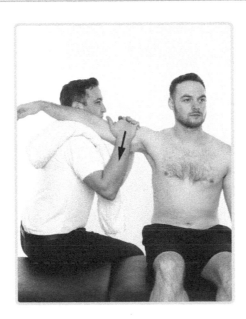

- The patient is in a seated position with the arm of the affected side raised to just above 90°; the patient's arm is positioned in abduction, with their elbow supported and in contact with the therapist's shoulder who is using a towel for added support and comfort.

- Stand in front of them on the affected side, in a lunge stance.

- Your contact hands are slightly inferior to the AC joint.

- The patient's elbow is being used as a fulcrum/pivot for the technique.

- Take up the skin slack and gain pre-tension by applying a gentle movement from superior to inferior.

- Once pre-tension has been taken up and the restricted barrier reached, the patient should inhale, and then on exhalation apply an HVLA in an oblique inferior direction.

Supine superior to inferior glenohumeral (GH) and acromioclavicular (AC) joint HVLA in abduction

- The patient is in a supine position with the arm of the affected side raised to just above 90°; the patient's arm is positioned in abduction.

- Stand in front of them on the affected side, in a lunge stance.

- Your outside arm locks and secures the patient's arm against their body, holding above the elbow – this is the supporting arm.

- Your contact hand is slightly inferior to the AC joint, either as a webbed hand or pisiform contact.

- The patient's arm is being used as a fulcrum/ pivot for the technique; by securing the arm, you can take it into abduction.

- Take up the skin slack and gain pre-tension by bringing the arm into abduction while applying an inferior HVLA in an inferior direction.

- Tip – once the patient's arm is secured, you can lean slightly away from the patient, adding an element of slight traction to the HVLA.

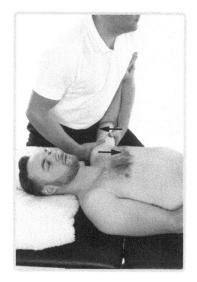

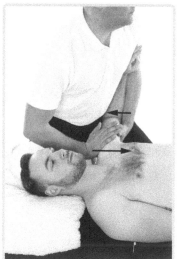

Pisiform hand contact or webbed hand contact

Supine anteroposterior glenohumeral (GH) and acromioclavicular (AC) joint HVLA in abduction

- The patient is in a supine position with the arm of the affected side raised to just above 90°; the patient's arm is positioned in abduction.

- Stand in front of them on the affected side, in a lunge stance.

- Your outside arm locks and secures the patient's arm against their anterior superior iliac spine (ASIS), holding above the elbow – this is the supporting arm.

- Your contact hand is slightly inferior to the AC joint, either as a pisiform contact or thenar hypothenar contact.

- The patient's arm is being used as a fulcrum/pivot for the technique; by securing the arm, you can take it into abduction.

- Take up the skin slack and gain pre-tension by bringing the arm into abduction while applying an HVLA in an anteroposterior direction.

- Tip – once the patient's arm is secured, you can lean slightly away from the patient, adding an element of slight traction to the HVLA.

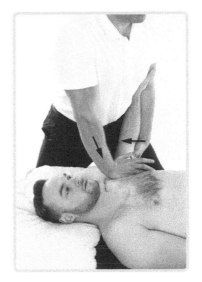

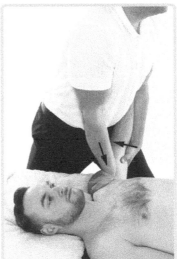

Pisiform hand contact or thenar hypothenar hand contact

Supine distal anteroposterior glenohumeral (GH) and acromioclavicular (AC) joint HVLA in abduction

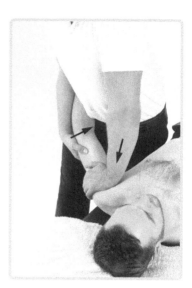

- The patient is in a supine position, with the arm of the affected side raised to just above 90°; the patient's arm is positioned in abduction.

- Stand in front of them on the affected side, in a lunge stance.

- Your outside arm locks and secures the patient's arm against their ASIS, holding above the elbow; this is the supporting arm leaning slightly away to induce slight traction.

- Your contact hand is slightly inferior to the AC joint.

- Take up the skin slack and gain pre-tension by maintaining distraction, applying gradual pressure, and once you have reached the barrier, apply a shallow anterior to posterior HVLA.

Seated clavicle lift technique

- This technique is applicable for the clavicle, and is a superior thrust technique.

- The patient is in a seated position with the arm of the affected side raised; position the patient's hand behind the back of the head and neck to support the cervical spine.

- Stand behind the patient.

- Contact the forearm of the patient with your hand, allowing your thumb to be positioned inferiorly to the clavicle; the thumb will sit underneath the clavicle (the first picture).

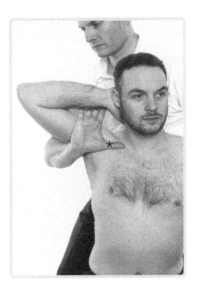

- Bring the patient's elbow down while maintaining contact with the forearm, and with the thumb still positioned underneath the clavicle (the second picture).

- Take up the skin slack and gain pre-tension by applying a superior movement upwards; once you have reached the barrier, apply a shallow superior HVLA, driving the clavicle upwards (the third picture).

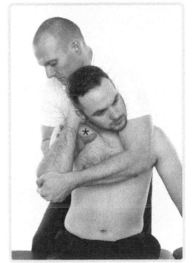

RIB MANIPULATION TECHNIQUES

Prone ipsilateral rib, R1-R3

- Stand on the affected side of the patient.

- With the left hand, locate the rib angle or costotransverse joint of the target segment.

- Use the right hand to contact the anterior aspect of the shoulder girdle.

- Using the right hand as the support hand, bring the shoulder posteriorly while applying direct compression anteriorly on the rib angle.

- Ask the patient to breathe deeply in, then out, following the rib as it drops away from your hand.

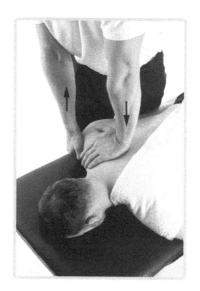

- At the end of the exhalation, apply a manipulation posteriorly-anteriorly (PA) towards the table.

Supine contra-lateral anterior rib, R1-R5

- Stand opposite the affected side of the patient.

- With the left hand, locate and contact the sternum and apply a stabilising compression.

- Use the right hand to contact the anterior rib angle.

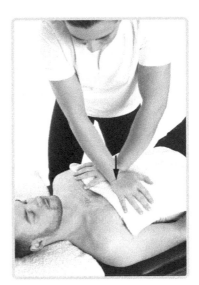

- Using the left hand as the support hand, apply pressure posteriorly while applying direct compression anteriorly on the rib angle with the other hand.

- Ask the patient to breathe deeply in, then out, following the rib as it drops away from your hand.

- At the end of the exhalation, apply a manipulation directly AP towards the table.

Prone 1st rib in extension

- Stand at the head of the patient.

- Get the patient to move their head into supported extension by resting their chin on the table, looking upwards; this locks out the cervical spine, protecting the vascular structures.

- Use side-bending and rotation to move the head into a locked position to direct the thrust towards the 1st rib, with the MCP joint of the driving hand in contact with the 1st rib, applying light pressure towards the opposite axilla.

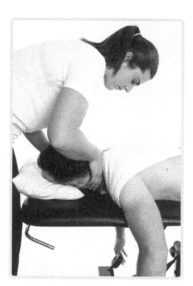

- Using your left hand as the support hand,
  bring the head into rotation while applying direct compression anteriorly on the rib angle.

- Ask the patient to breathe deeply in, then out, following the rib as it drops away from your hand.

- At the end of the exhalation, apply a manipulation by bilaterally rotating the head towards the left hand and driving obliquely towards the opposite axilla.

Supine contra-lateral posterior rib rotation, R3-R6

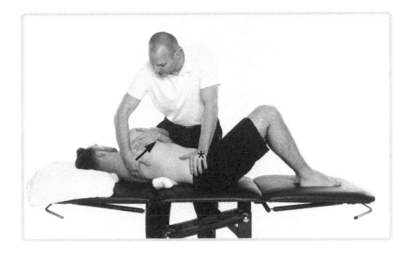

- The patient lies supine, with the legs bent, feet placed on the table to aid as a fulcrum.

- The patient's arms should be folded across the chest.

- Stand at the patient's unaffected side and adopt an asymmetrical stance.

- With the heel of your dominant contact hand, contact the patient's contra lateral ASIS, bracing the ASIS against the table.

- With the other hand, grasp the patient's posterior shoulder, superior and lateral to the scapula.

- Ask the patient to inhale and exhale.

- Towards the end of exhalation, bring the ribs into rotation building the pre-tension; as the barrier is reached, apply a rotation thrust towards you, stabilising the ASIS to ensure no movement through the pelvis.

Supine contra-lateral posterior rib manipulation, R1-R6

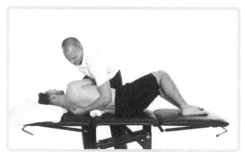 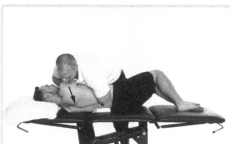

- The patient lies supine, with the legs bent, feet placed on the table to aid as a fulcrum.

- The patient's contra-lateral arm should be either folded across the chest or holding the opposite shoulder for stability; a small towel can be placed under the patient to increase slight extension into the thoracic spine.

- Adopt an asymmetrical stance with your lead leg contacting the table.

- Rotate the patient towards you, and, using a flat palm with a thenar eminence, contact against the target rib; for ribs 1–3 bring the hand higher.

- With the other hand, grasp the patient's posterior shoulder girdle and lock it against your chest; apply compression at an oblique angle towards the rib.

- Ask the patient to inhale and exhale.

- Towards the end of exhalation, lean towards the ribs, building the pre-tension; as the barrier is reached, apply an oblique thrust away from you.

Seated posterior rib manipulation, R1-R4

- The patient is seated with the therapist standing behind them.

- The patient's arms should be folded across the chest. Brace the patient's non-affected side with your sternum. The picture shows the therapist's left hand holding onto the patient's elbows – this will allow the therapist to pull them into thoracic extension.

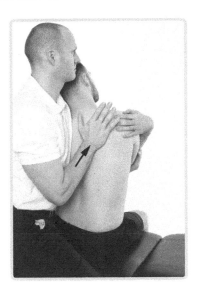

- Adopt an asymmetrical stance with your lead leg contacting the table.

- Extend the patient towards you, and, using a flat palm with a thenar eminence, contact against the target rib; for ribs 1–3, bring the hand higher.

- With the other hand, at the same time bring the patient into slight extension; this will allow you to build up the pre-tension.

- Ask the patient to inhale and exhale.

- Towards the end of exhalation, with the right hand apply a thrust in a superior anterior oblique angle while bringing the patient into extension.

Seated posterior rib manipulation sternum contact, R2-R4

- The patient is seated with the therapist standing behind them.

- The picture shows the patient's right arm placed behind their head with their left hand secured across their chest. Brace the patient's non-affected side with your sternum. The picture shows the therapist's left hand holding onto the patient's elbow – this will allow the therapist to pull them into thoracic extension; the therapist's right hand has looped under the patient's to contact the forearm.

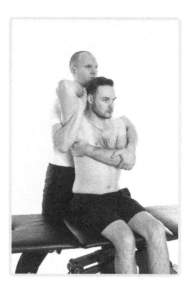

- Adopt an asymmetrical stance with your lead leg contacting the table.

- Extend the patient towards you, using your sternum to contact against the target rib.

- As you pull your right hand backwards, apply an oblique drive with your sternum anterior and superior; this helps bring the patient into slight extension, and will allow you to build up the pre-tension by taking out the tissue slack.

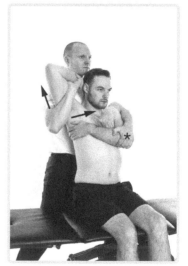

- Ask the patient to inhale and exhale.

- Towards the end of exhalation, with the sternum apply a thrust in a superior anterior oblique angle while bringing the patient into extension.

7

ELBOW, WRIST AND HAND

Introduction

Manipulative therapy is a popular treatment modality for managing a broad spectrum of upper extremity conditions (Brantingham *et al.* 2013). Studies have reported patient improvement with manipulative interventions in various upper extremity problems, ranging from carpal tunnel syndrome to lateral epicondylitis and cubital tunnel syndrome, among others (Brantingham *et al.* 2013; Lawrence 2016; Salehi *et al.* 2015; Saunders *et al.* 2016). The non-invasive treatment approaches used in manipulative therapy of the elbow, wrist and hand make it an attractive option for many patients (Saunders *et al.* 2016).

The therapeutic goal of the diverse manipulative techniques applied to the elbow, wrist and hand is to minimise patient discomfort while yielding the best treatment results. Many manipulative treatments of the upper extremity reduce inflammation, alleviate spasticity, correct bone misalignment, reduce force overload, promote rapid healing and ultimately result in increased upper extremity potency, tenacity and flexibility (Saunders *et al.* 2016).

This chapter will serve as a helpful resource to therapists as they assist patients presenting with various pathological conditions of the elbow, wrist and hand. Anatomical information on the various joints of the upper extremity and their associated ranges of motion are highlighted to give readers a high-level overview of the normal mobility of the upper limb. Common injuries of the elbow, wrist and hand, along with special tests for detecting pathological conditions of the upper limb, are also outlined. The chapter also includes a section on red flag symptoms to help therapists diagnose potentially serious pathologies early and avert adverse treatment effects.

Joints

The elbow joint forms a mechanical connection between the shoulder and the hand (see Table 7.1). The joint is a typical composite articulation, being formed by the joining of the lower end of the humerus with the upper ends of the radius and ulna. The joint thus consists of three articulations that include the humeroulnar joint, humeroradial joint and radioulnar joint. These three articulations share a mutual articular capsule, which is generous and relaxed, particularly ventrally and dorsally (OpenStax 2018). The humeroradial portion of the elbow joint involves the capitulum of the humerus with the depressed distal surface on the head of the radius. The humeroradial articulation is not involved in the hinge movement at the elbow, since the ends of the respective bones are scarcely in contact during flexion. The humeroradial articulation is only passively involved in the pivot movement of the proximal radioulnar joint, since the radius rotates in the socket about its long axis, and the actual pivot movement takes place in the proximal and distal radioulnar articulations. The major functions of the elbow include support for the forearm and affording fine movements of the hand and wrist (Standring 2016).

In contrast, the hand is composed of carpals, metacarpals and phalanges. The radius and ulnar meet at the hand to form the wrist. The functions of these include object handling, providing oppositional grip, communicating and various other tasks in daily life (Standring 2016).

Table 7.1. Joints of the elbow, wrist and hand

Joint name	Description	Function
Elbow joint	• A complex synovial hinge joint • Formed between the distal end of the humerus in the upper arm and the proximal ends of the ulnar and radius in the forearm • Comprises three distinct articulations, namely, the humeroulnar joint, humeroradial joint and superior radioulnar joint • Bounded by a single fibrous capsule that encircles the entire joint complex	• Permits flexion and extension of the forearm in the sagittal plane around the coronal axis • Allows rotation of the forearm and the wrist
Humeroulnar/ olecron joint	• A modified diarthrodial joint • Formed between the junction of the trochlear notch of the ulnar and the trochlea of the humerus bones • Involves articulation between the humerus and ulna	• Allows for movements of flexion, extension and circumduction
Humeroradial joint	• A ball-and-socket joint • Formed where the capitulum of the humeral articulates with the fovea of the head of the radius	• Allows flexion and extension of the elbow with rotation of the radial head on the capitellum
Superior radioulnar joint	• A pivot joint enclosed within the elbow's articular tissue • Formed by an articulation between the head of the radius and radial notch of the ulnar	• Responsible for pronation and supination of the forearm

Joint name	Description	Function
Radiocarpal joint	• An ellipsoid synovial joint • Formed by the proximal row of the carpal bone except the pisiform, proximally by the distal end of the radius and the articular disc	• Aids in stability of the wrist • Permits the wrist to move along two axes • Supports flexion, extension, adduction and abduction of the wrist
Intercarpal joints	• Synovial joints • Form articulations between the individual carpal bones • Subdivided into three sets of articulations: joints of the proximal row and distal row and joints between these two • Carpal bones united with anterior, posterior and interosseous ligaments	• Contribute to total wrist mobility
Midcarpal joint	• A synovial joint • Formed by eight carpal bones to make the carpus • Also formed between the proximal and distal carpal rows • Composed of a very extensive and irregular joint cavity	• Allows augmentation of movements at the wrist joint • Movements include flexion, extension, abduction and adduction of the wrist
Carpometa-carpal joints	• Synovial joints formed between the distal row of carpal bones and the proximal row of five metacarpal bones • Reinforced by three main ligaments including the anterior oblique, first intermetacarpal and posterior oblique ligaments	• Permit flexion and extension in the plane of the palm of the hand, abduction and adduction in a plane at right angles to the palm, circumduction and opposition
Intermetacarpal joints	• Plane synovial joints • Formed between the bases of the 2nd to 5th metacarpal bones • Contain a fibrous capsule that gives them stability • Strengthened by a group of ligaments, including the dorsal, palmar and interosseous metacarpal ligaments	• Permit slight gliding movements • Allow for some flexion-extension and adjunct rotation
Metacarpo-phalangeal joints	• Condyloid joints • Connect the distal head of metacarpals to the proximal phalanges of the fingers • Supported by several ligaments, including the palmar and collateral	• Allow movement of the fingers in different directions including flexion-extension, abduction-adduction and circumduction

Interphalangeal joints	• Uniaxial hinge joints	• Allow flexion and extension movements
	• Formed between the phalanges of the fingers	
	• Connect the heads of the phalanges to the bases of the next distal phalanges	
	• Subdivided into two sets of articulations: proximal interphalangeal joints and distal interphalangeal joints	
	• Ligaments include palmar and collateral ligaments that provide stability	

Sources: OpenStax (2018); Standring (2016)

Range of motion

The elbow joint allows for flexion-extension and pronation-supination movements (see Tables 7.2 and 7.3). Daily activities are allowed by minimum flexion and extension in combination with considerable pronation and supination (Zwerus *et al.* 2017).

The elbow joint is a complex hinge involving three separate articulations that include the humeroulnar joint, humeroradial joint and radioulnar joint (Standring 2016). The three articulations comprise a single compound joint and coordinate to allow for movements such as flexion and extension of the upper arm as well as supination and pronation of the forearm and wrist (Villaseñor-Ovies *et al.* 2012).

Table 7.2. Normal range of motion of the elbow joint

Movement type	Range of motion
Flexion	130–154°
Extension	6–11°
Pronation	75–85°
Supination	80–104°

Sources: Soucie et al. (2011); Zwerus et al. (2017)

Table 7.3. Minimum range of motion of the elbow for activities of daily living

Movement type	Range of motion
Flexion	130°
Extension	30°
Pronation	50°
Supination	50°

Source: Zwerus et al. *(2017)*

The wrist joint allows for movement along two axes, thus permitting flexion, extension, adduction and abduction (see Tables 7.4 and 7.5). The hand also encompasses an incredible range of motion (see Table 7.6). The range of motion for the two joints, in conjunction with the muscles of the forearm, consequently allows various activities to be achieved.

Table 7.4. Normal range of motion of the wrist

Movement type	Range of motion
Flexion	60–80°
Extension	60–75°
Radial deviation	20–25°
Ulnar deviation	30–39°

Source: Norkin and White (2017)

Table 7.5. Functional and mean range of motion of the wrist in activities of daily living

Motion unit	Range of motion
Functional range of motion in activities of daily living	<ul><li>45° of flexion</li><li>50° of extension</li><li>15° of radial deviation</li><li>40° of ulnar deviation</li></ul>
Mean range of motion in activities of daily living	<ul><li>50° of flexion</li><li>51° of extension</li><li>12° of radial deviation</li><li>40° of ulnar deviation</li></ul>

Sources: Brigstocke et al. *(2013); Nelson* et al. *(1994)*

Table 7.6. Normal range of motion of the finger joints

Joint name	Motion type	Average
Metacarpophalangeal joint	Flexion	90–100°
	Extension	20–45°
Proximal interphalangeal joint	Flexion	90–120°
	Extension	0°
Distal interphalangeal joint	Flexion	70–90°
	Extension	0°
Metacarpophalangeal joint (thumb)	Flexion	50–60°
	Extension	14–23°
Interphalangeal joint (thumb)	Flexion	67–80°
Carpometacarpal joint (thumb)	Flexion	15–45°
	Extension	0–20°
	Abduction	50–70°

Source: Norkin and White (2017)

Common injuries

Upper extremity injuries are common to all age groups of both sexes. The injuries include traumatic and chronic over-use-type damages while others depend on specific occupational demands. Falls, motor vehicle accidents, violent activities, sports accidents or penetrating trauma are also causes of major injuries to the elbow, wrist and hand (Dines *et al.* 2015). Such injuries can lead to substantial disability and negatively affect regular activities of life. The injuries may damage both bony and soft tissue and may require surgery, hence affecting return to duty and work readiness for those in various occupations such as the military and in the mechanical industries (Blackwell *et al.* 2014) One common injury includes carpal tunnel syndrome and this is most often treated surgically (see Table 7.7).

Commonly encountered conditions of the upper extremity include rotator cuff injury, internal impingement, superior labral tears and epicondylitis of the elbow (Dines *et al.* 2015). Such injuries are common in sports such as tennis, squash and badminton that involve overhead arm motions. The greatest number of injuries is observed in the wrist (15.2% of all upper extremity injuries) and the digits of the hand (38.4% of all injuries) (Bachoura, Ferikes and Lubahn 2017; Ootes, Lambers and Ring 2012).

Table 7.7. Common injuries of the elbow, wrist and hand

Common injuries	Incidence	Characteristics
Dislocation of the radial head or pulled elbow	• 50,000 cases annually (UK) • 6–13 cases per 100,000 people (USA)	• An upper extremity injury • Due to a pulling force on the extended elbow joint and pronated forearm • Results in radial head subluxation or entrapment of the annular ligament of the radius in the humeroradial joint in children under 5 years • Has a slight predominance in girls and on the left hand
Lateral epicondylitis	• 4–7 cases per 1000 people annually (UK) • 2.98 per 1000 person-years (USA)	• An over-use injury of wrist extensor musculature, i.e., extensor carpi radialis brevis • Due to repetitive strain from tasks and activities that involve loaded and repeated gripping, wrist extension, radial deviation and/or forearm supination • Common in people above 40 years • Lateral epicondyle of the humerus becomes sore and tender • With an acute or chronic inflammation and micro-tearing of fibres in the extensor tendons
Olecranon bursitis	• Not reported	• Inflammation of the bursa • Due to trauma, prolonged pressure, infection, leading to bleeding within the bursa and release of inflammatory mediators • Pain, swelling and redness near the olecranon process • Affects men between the ages of 30 and 60 years
Wrist bone fracture (scaphoid)	• 12.4 in 100,000 people annually (UK) • 20,000 individuals annually (USA)	• Fracture of the carpal bone • Common in sports involving high-impact injuries • Predominant in men • Due to falls on an outstretched hand, athletic injury or motor vehicle accident • Characterised by pain and tenderness in the area just below the base of the thumb

Mallet finger	• 1–2% of the adult population (UK) • 5.6% of all tendinous lesions in the hand and wrist (USA)	• A traumatic zone I lesion of the extensor tendon with either tendon rapture or bony evulsion at the base of the distal phalanx • Common in young men • Usually occurs when an axial load is applied to a straight digit tip followed by extreme distal interphalangeal joint hyperflexion or hyperextension • Characterised by tenderness, pain, swelling and inability to straighten the tip of that finger, reduced dexterity, decreased pinch strength and grasp capability
De Quervain syndrome	• 2.8 per 1000 person-years (women) (USA) • 0.6 per 1000 person-years (men) (USA)	• A condition affecting the tendons on the thumb • Due to repetitive hand and wrist movement • Predominant in middle-aged women • Symptoms include difficulty gripping, pain and tenderness on certain movements of the wrist and pain near the base of the thumb • Peak prevalence among those in their 40s and 50s
Carpal tunnel syndrome	• 27.68 per 10,000 people per year (UK) • 1.5–3.5 per 1000 person-years (USA)	• Most common entrapment mononeuropathy • Characterised by compression of the median nerve as it passes through the fibro-osseous tunnel beneath the flexor retinaculum • Due to forceful or repetitive hand and wrist movements • Prevalent in middle-aged (30–60 years age group) obese women • Prone groups may be having myxoedema, acromegaly, pregnancy, obesity, rheumatoid arthritis, primary amyloidosis or tophaceous gout • Symptoms include numbness, tingling, pain and weakness in the palm of the hand and fingers

Sources: Alla, Deal and Dempsey (2014); Bachoura et al. (2017); Becker, McCormick and Renfrew (2008); Blackwell et al. (2014); Burton et al. (2018); Daly et al. (2018); Dines et al. (2015); Garala, Taub and Dias (2016); Gobbi et al. (2017); Halstead and Bernhardt (2017); Heydari et al. (2018); Irie et al. (2014); Robertson et al. (2018); Salazar Botero et al. (2016); Sanders et al. (2015); Vitello et al. (2014); Wolf, Mountcastle and Owens (2009); Wolf et al. (2010)

Red flags

Red flag symptoms aid in the early detection of potentially serious pathology patients (see Table 7.8). When a red flag symptom is identified, the therapist should use sound clinical reasoning and exercise great caution to minimise the risk of adverse outcomes from the treatment (WHO 2005).

Table 7.8. Red flags for serious pathology in the elbow, wrist and hand

Condition	Signs and symptoms
Compartment syndrome	• History of blunt trauma, crush injury or surgery • Continual pain and tension in the forearm • Pain that increases with stretching of affected muscles • Involved compartment feels tender and tense on physical examination • Weakened pulse and protracted capillary refill • Paraesthesia (tingling or pins and needles sensation), paresis and sensory deficits
Colles' fracture	• Recent fall onto an outstretched arm with high-impact wrist extension • Pain when attempting to extend the wrist • Young male or older female • Inflammation of the wrist • Wrist kept in a neutral position
Radial head fracture	• Recent fall onto an outstretched arm • Tenderness of the radial head • Elbow joint effusion (affected arm is retained in a loose packed position) • Constrained or excruciating supination and pronation active range of motion
Raynaud's phenomenon	• A family history of the phenomenon • Woman undergoing oestrogen therapy • Exposure to extreme cold and associated frostbite injury • Underlying collagen vascular disease • Hyperaemic erythema and/or cyanosis of the fingers • Taking medical drugs promoting vasoconstriction (e.g., B-blockers, amphetamines, decongestants, caffeine)
Avascular necrosis	• Slow onset of pain, with upper arm stiffness • History of alcohol and oral steroid abuse • History of cancer treatment (especially chemotherapy)
Reflex sympathetic dystrophy or complex regional pain syndrome	• History of trauma or surgical treatment • Severe burning/aching pain disproportionate to the stimulus • Pain not controlled with common analgesics • Evidence of secondary hyperalgesia/hypersensitivity • Affected area appears inflamed and with a large temperature difference between involved and uninvolved limbs

Lunate dislocation or fracture	• Pain in the wrist area, especially at wrist extension end ranges
	• History of falling onto an extended hand or a dorsiflexion injury of the hand
	• Severe pain with gripping things or moving the wrist
	• Decreased grip strength and/or pain when grasping objects
Scaphoid fracture	• History of falling onto an extended hand
	• Prevalent in males (15–30 years old) and females with osteoporosis
	• Wrist inflammation and/or bruising
	• Pain with or without swelling or bruising at the base of the thumb
	• Tenderness over scaphoid tubercle
	• Pain intensified with grasping objects
	• Movement limitations of the wrist or thumb
Long flexor tendon rupture	• Injury on the palmar side of the hand
	• Sensory limitations of the fingertip region
	• Forceful flexor contraction
	• Lacerations in tendon area
	• Loss of isolated distal interphalangeal (DIP) joint or proximal interphalangeal (PIP) joint flexion (active)
	• Vigorous flexor contraction
	• Possible palpable defect in affected muscle
Melanoma	• History of malignancy
	• Female <40 years of age or male >40 years of age
	• Fair skin
	• History of sunburn
	• Asymmetric/irregular-shaped lesion with notched borders
	• Inexplicable deformity, mass or swelling with uneven colour and a diameter >6mm
	• Sudden, unplanned weight loss
	• Extreme exhaustion
	• Constant or intermittent low-grade fever
Space infection of the hand	• Heightened fever, chills and general malaise
	• Recent history of infection (e.g., urinary tract or skin infection)
	• Recent history of lacerations, bruising or puncture wound (human or animal bite)
	• Lack of appetite
	• Kanavel cardinal signs (digit flexion, uniform swelling, tenderness of involved tendon sheath, excruciating pain on attempted hyperextension)

Sources: Boissonnault (2005); Godges (no date); Mabvuure et al. (2012); Prasarn and Ouellette (2011); Saunders et al. (2016); Skirven et al. (2011)

Special tests

Table 7.9 is not an exhaustive list of special tests but gives you, the therapist, a guide for this area. If you are unsure of the interpretation of any test that you complete with your patient, we advise that you refer to the most appropriate medical professional for further investigations.

Table 7.9. Special tests for elbow, wrist and hand dysfunction

Test	Procedure	Positive sign	Interpretation	Test statistics
Adduction/ varus stress test	The patient sits with their elbow in slight flexion. While stabilising the upper arm medially with one hand, the therapist adducts the patient's forearm in the elbow joint, creating varus stress to the lateral collateral ligament	• Lateral pain with or without an increase in laxity when compared with the uninvolved elbow	✓ Lateral collateral ligament injury (varus instability)	Not reported
Valgus stress test	The seated patient's elbow is placed in 20–30° of flexion. The therapist ensures that the patient's forearm is supinated before applying valgus stress to the elbow	• No firm end point is palpated • Reproduction of patient's pain	✓ Medial collateral ligament instability	Specificity: 0.60 Sensitivity: 0.66
Tennis elbow sign/ Thomson test	The standing patient is instructed to make a fist while extending the elbow. The therapist should ensure the patient's hand is in slight dorsiflexion before immobilising the dorsal wrist with one hand and grasping the fist with the other hand The patient then extends their fist against the therapist's resistance. The last step may also be achieved with the therapist pressing the dorsiflexed fist into flexion against the patient's resistance	• Intense pain over the lateral epicondyle and lateral extensor compartment	✓ Lateral epicondylitis	Not reported

Test	Procedure	Signs	Indication	Reliability
Tinel's sign test	Elbow: With the patient seated, the therapist grasps the upper arm and gently taps on the ulnar nerve groove with a reflex hammer Wrist: The therapist slightly dorsiflexes the patient's hand with the dorsum of the wrist resting on a cushion on the table. The therapist, using a reflex hammer or an index finger, gently taps the median nerve at the wrist crease	• Pain after gentle tapping of the ulnar nerve groove • Paraesthesia distal to the point of pressure and pain radiating into the hand	✓ Elbow: Cubital tunnel syndrome; ulnar nerve compression neuropathy ✓ Wrist: Median nerve lesion: tenosynovitis; carpal tunnel syndrome	Elbow Specificity: 0.98 Sensitivity: 0.70 Wrist Specificity: 0.77 Sensitivity: 0.50
Phalen test (wrist flexion sign)	The patient drops their hands into palmar flexion while pressing the dorsa of the hands. The patient holds the position for 1–2 minutes Pressing the dorsa of the hands would increase carpal tunnel pressure	• Intense paraesthesia in the area innervated by the median nerve	✓ Median nerve damage ✓ Carpal tunnel syndrome ✓ Tenosynovitis ✓ Pronator syndrome	Specificity: 0.73 Sensitivity: 0.68
Murphy's test	The patient is instructed to make a fist and the therapist observes the position of the 3rd metacarpal	• 3rd metacarpal level with the 2nd and 4th metacarpals	✓ Lunate dislocation	Specificity: 0.54 Sensitivity: 0.49
Flexor digitorum superficialis test	The patient is instructed to flex the proximal interphalangeal joint of the affected finger. The therapist keeps the other fingers in extension	• Lack of proximal interphalangeal joint flexion	✓ Flexor digitorum superficialis tendon no longer intact ✓ Tenosynovitis (only when pain is present)	Specificity: 0.72 Sensitivity: 1.0
Flexor digitorum profundus test or sweater/ jersey finger sign	The therapist places their index and middle fingers on the volar aspects of the patient's involved finger, keeping the proximal interphalangeal joint in extension. The patient is then instructed to flex the distal interphalangeal joint	• Difficulty in flexing the distal interphalangeal joint	✓ Torn flexor digitorum profundus tendon ✓ Tenosynovitis (only when pain is present)	Not reported

Test	Procedure	Positive sign	Interpretation	Test statistics
Allen's test/ fist closure test	The seated patient is instructed to raise their arm above the horizontal plane. The therapist, while holding the patient's wrist, applies finger pressure to compress the radial and ulnar arteries The patient is then instructed to clench a tight fist for 1 minute to squeeze venous blood out of the hand via the posterior veins. When the time has lapsed, the patient lowers the arm and relaxes the now pale hand. The therapist releases compression one artery at a time, while observing the colour of the hand and fingers	• Slow recession of ischaemic changes in the hand	✓ Compromised radial or ulnar artery	Specificity: 0.97 Sensitivity: 0.73

Sources: Buckup and Buckup (2016); Dhatt and Prabhakar (2019); Karbach and Elfar (2017); Magee (2014); Pandey et al. *(2014); Physical Therapists (no date); Valdés-Flores* et al. *(2019); Wald, Mendoza and Mihm (2019); Zwerus* et al. *(2018)*

References

Alla, S.R., Deal, N.D. and Dempsey, I.J. (2014) 'Current concepts: Mallet finger.' *Hand* 9(2), 138–144. doi:10.1007/s11552-014-9609-y

Bachoura, A., Ferikes, A.J. and Lubahn, J.D. (2017) 'A review of mallet finger and jersey finger injuries in the athlete.' *Current Reviews in Musculoskeletal Medicine* 10(1), 1–9. doi:10.1007/s12178-017-9395-6

Becker, G.E., McCormick, F.M. and Renfrew, M.J. (2008) 'Methods of milk expression for lactating women.' *Cochrane Database of Systematic Reviews*. doi:10.1002/14651858.CD006170.pub2

Blackwell, J.R., Hay, B.A., Bolt, A.M. and Hay, S.M. (2014) 'Olecranon bursitis: A systematic overview.' *Shoulder & Elbow* 6(3), 182–190. doi:10.1177/1758573214532787

Boissonnault, W.G. (2005) *Primary Care for the Physical Therapist*. St Louis, MO: Elsevier Saunders. doi:10.1016/B978-0-7216-9659-1.X5001-1

Brantingham, J.W., Cassa, T.K., Bonnefin, D., Pribicevic, M., Robb, A., Pollard, H. *et al.* (2013) 'Manipulative and multimodal therapy for upper extremity and temporomandibular disorders: A systematic review.' *Journal of Manipulative and Physiological Therapeutics* 36(3), 143–201. doi:10.1016/j.jmpt.2013.04.001

Brigstocke, G., Hearnden, A., Holt, C.A. and Whatling, G. (2013) 'The functional range of movement of the human wrist.' *Journal of Hand Surgery (European Volume)* 38(5), 554–556. doi:10.1177/1753193412458751

Buckup, K. and Buckup, J. (2016) *Clinical Tests for the Musculoskeletal System: Examinations, Signs, Phenomena*. 3rd edn. Stuttgart: Thieme Medical Publishers.

Burton, C.L., Chen, Y., Chesterton, L.S. and van der Windt, D.A. (2018) 'Trends in the prevalence, incidence and surgical management of carpal tunnel syndrome between 1993 and 2013: An observational analysis of UK primary care records.' *British Medical Journal Open* 8(6), e020166. doi:10.1136/bmjopen-2017-020166

Daly, C.A., Boden, A.L., Hutton, W.C. and Gottschalk, M.B. (2018) 'Biomechanical strength of retrograde fixation in proximal third scaphoid fractures.' *Hand*. doi:10.1177/1558944718769385

Dhatt, S.S. and Prabhakar, S. (eds) (2019) *Handbook of Clinical Examination in Orthopedics*. Singapore: Springer Singapore. doi:10.1007/978-981-13-1235-9

Dines, J.S., Bedi, A., Williams, P.N., Dodson, C.C., Ellenbecker, T.S., Altcheck, D.W. *et al.* (2015) 'Tennis injuries: Epidemiology.' *The Journal of the American Academy of Orthopaedic Surgeons* 23(3), 181–189. doi:10.5435/JAAOS-D-13-00148

Garala, K., Taub, N.A. and Dias, J.J. (2016) 'The epidemiology of fractures of the scaphoid.' *The Bone & Joint Journal* 98-B(5), 654–659. doi:10.1302/0301-620X.98B5.36938

Gobbi, A., Espregueira-Mendes, J., Lane, J.G. and Karahan, M. (eds) (2017) *Bio-orthopaedics*. Berlin, Heidelberg: Springer. doi:10.1007/978-3-662-54181-4

Godges, J. (no date) 'Red Flags for Potential Serious Conditions in Patients with Elbow, Wrist, or Hand Problems.' Kaiser Permanente Southern California Physiotherapy Residency. Available at https://s3-us-west-2.amazonaws.com/scal-assets/scal-pt-residencyfellowship/03ElbowReg ion/01MedicalScreening-Elbow,WristandHandRegion.pdf

Halstead, M.E. and Bernhardt, D.T. (2017) 'Elbow Dislocation.' *eMedicine*. Available at https://emedicine.medscape.com/article/96758-overview

Heydari, F., Shariat, S.S., Majidinejad, S. and Masoumi, B. (2018) 'The use of ultrasonography for the confirmation of pulled elbow treatment.' *Journal of Emergency Practice and Trauma* 4(1), 24–28. doi:10.15171/jept.2017.24

Irie, T., Sono, T., Hayama, Y., Matsumoto, T. and Matsushita, M. (2014) 'Investigation on 2331 cases of pulled elbow over the last 10 years.' *Pediatric Reports* 6(2), 26–28. doi:10.4081/pr.2014.5090

Karbach, L.E. and Elfar, J. (2017) 'Elbow instability: Anatomy, biomechanics, diagnostic maneuvers, and testing.' *The Journal of Hand Surgery* 42(2), 118–126. doi:10.1016/j.jhsa.2016.11.025

Lawrence, D. (2016) 'Chiropractic for the treatment of disease.' *Focus on Alternative and Complementary Therapies* 21(1), 46–47. doi:10.1111/fct.12223

Mabvuure, N.T., Malahlas, M., Hindocha, S., Khan, W. and Juma, A. (2012) 'Acute compartment syndrome of the limbs: Current concepts and management.' *The Open Orthopaedics Journal* 6, 535–543. doi:10.2174/1874325001206010535

Magee, D.J. (2014) *Orthopedic Physical Assessment*. 6th edn. St Louis, MO: Saunders.

Nelson, D.L., Mitchell, M.A., Groszewski, P.G., Pennick, S.L. and Manske, P.R. (1994) 'Wrist Range of Motion in Activities of Daily Living.' in F. Schuind, K.N. An, W.P. Cooney III and M. Garcia-Elias (eds) *Advances in the Biomechanics of the Hand and Wrist*. Boston, MA: Springer US. doi:10.1007/978-1-4757-9107-5_29

Norkin, C.C. and White, D.J. (2017) *Measurement of Joint Motion: A Guide to Goniometry*. 5th edn. Philadelphia, PA: F.A. Davis Company.

Ootes, D., Lambers, K.T. and Ring, D.C. (2012) 'The epidemiology of upper extremity injuries presenting to the Emergency Department in the United States.' *Hand* 7(1), 18–22. doi:10.1007/s11552-011-9383-z

OpenStax (2018) *Anatomy and Physiology*. OpenStax CNX. Available at http://cnx.org/contents/14fb4ad7-39a1-4eee-ab6e-3ef2482e3e22@12.8

Pandey, T., Slaughter, A.J., Reynolds, K.A., Jambhekar, K., David, R.M. and Hasan, S.A. (2014) 'Clinical orthopedic examination findings in the upper extremity: Correlation with imaging studies and diagnostic efficacy.' *RadioGraphics* 34(2), e24–e40. doi:10.1148/rg.342125061

Physical Therapists (no date) *Orthopedic Special Tests: Upper Extremity*. Available at https://pdhtherapy.com/wp-content/uploads/2016/09/PROOF6_PDH_OrthopedicSpecialTests_UPPER-Extremity_StandAloneCourse.pdf

Prasarn, M.L. and Ouellette, E.A. (2011) 'Acute compartment syndrome of the upper extremity.' *The Journal of the American Academy of Orthopaedic Surgeons 19*(1), 49–58. Available at www.ncbi.nlm.nih.gov/pubmed/21205767

Robertson, G.A.J., Ang, K.K., Maffulli, N., Keenan, G. and Wood, A.M. (2018) 'Return to sport following Lisfranc injuries: A systematic review and meta-analysis.' *Foot and Ankle Surgery 10*(2), 101–114. doi:10.1016/j.fas.2018.07.008

Salazar Botero, S., Hidalgo Diaz, J.J., Benaïda, A., Collon, S., Facca, S. and Liverneaux, P.A. (2016) 'Review of acute traumatic closed mallet finger injuries in adults.' *Archives of Plastic Surgery 43*(2), 134–144. doi:10.5999/aps.2016.43.2.134

Salehi, A., Hashemi, N., Imanieh, M.H. and Saber, M. (2015) 'Chiropractic: Is it efficient in treatment of diseases? Review of systematic reviews.' *International Journal of Community-based Nursing and Midwifery 3*(4), 244–54. Available at www.ncbi.nlm.nih.gov/pubmed/26448951

Sanders, T.L., Maradit Kremers, H., Bryan, A.J., Ransom, J.E., Smith, J. and Morrey, B.F. (2015) 'The epidemiology and health care burden of tennis elbow: A population-based study.' *The American Journal of Sports Medicine 43*(5), 1066–1071. doi:10.1177/0363546514568087

Saunders, R.J. Jr, Astifidis, R., Burke, S.L., Higgins, J. McClinton, M.A. (2016) *Hand and Upper Extremity Rehabilitation*. 4th edn. London: Churchill Livingstone. doi:10.1016/C2012-0-00728-4

Skirven, T.M., Osterman, A.L., Fedorczyk, J. and Amadio, P.C. (2011) *Rehabilitation of the Hand and Upper Extremity*, 2-Volume Set. 6th edn. Philadelphia, PA: Elsevier. Available at www.us.elsevierhealth.com/rehabilitation-of-the-hand-and-upper-extremity-2-volume-set-9780323056021.html#panel1

Soucie, J.M., Wang, C., Forsyth, A., Funk, S., Denny, M., Roach, K.E. *et al.* (2011) 'Range of motion measurements: Reference values and a database for comparison studies.' *Haemophilia 17*(3), 500–507. doi:10.1111/j.1365-2516.2010.02399.x

Standring, S. (ed.) (2016) *Gray's Anatomy: The Anatomical Basis of Clinical Practice*. 41st edn. New York: Elsevier. Available at www.elsevier.com/books/grays-anatomy/standring/978-0-7020-5230-9

Valdés-Flores, E., García-Álvarez, E., Garcí-Pérez, M.M., Castro-Govea, Y., Santos-Ibarra, A., Chacón-Martínez, H. *et al.* (2019) 'A test for the clinical evaluation of the flexor digitorum superficialis of the fifth finger.' *Annals of Plastic Surgery 82*(2), 166–168. doi:10.1097/SAP.0000000000001741

Villaseñor-Ovies, P., Vargas, A., Chiapas-Gasca, K., Canoso, J.J., Hernández-Díaz, C., Saavedra, M.A. *et al.* (2012) 'Clinical anatomy of the elbow and shoulder.' *Reumatología Clínica 8*, 13–24. doi:10.1016/j.reuma.2012.10.009

Vitello, S., Dvorkin, R., Sattler, S., Levy, D. and Ung, L. (2014) 'Epidemiology of nursemaid's elbow.' *Western Journal of Emergency Medicine 15*(4), 554–557. doi:10.5811/westjem.2014.1.20813

Wald, S.H., Mendoza, J. and Mihm, F.G. (2019) 'Procedures for vascular access.' *A Practice of Anesthesia for Infants and Children*, 1129–1145.e5. doi:10.1016/B978-0-323-42974-0.00049-5

WHO (World Health Organization) (2005) WHO *Guidelines on Basic Training and Safety in Chiropractic*. Geneva: WHO.

Wolf, J.M., Mountcastle, S. and Owens, B.D. (2009) 'Incidence of carpal tunnel syndrome in the US military population.' *Hand 4*(3), 289–293. doi:10.1007/s11552-009-9166-y

Wolf, J.M., Mountcastle, S., Burks, R., Sturdivant, R.X. and Owens, B.D. (2010) 'Epidemiology of lateral and medial epicondylitis in a military population.' *Military Medicine 175*(5), 336–339. Available at www.ncbi.nlm.nih.gov/pubmed/20486505

Zwerus, E.L., Somford, M.P., Maissan, F., Heisen, J., Eygendaal, D. and van den Bekerom, M.P. (2018) 'Physical examination of the elbow, what is the evidence? A systematic literature review.' *British Journal of Sports Medicine 52*(19), 1253–1260. doi:10.1136/bjsports-2016-096712

Zwerus, E.L., Willigenburg, N.W., Scholtes, V.A., Somford, M.P., Eygendaal, D. and van den Bekerom, M.P. (2017) 'Normative values and affecting factors for the elbow range of motion.' *Shoulder & Elbow* 11(3), 1–10. doi:10.1177/1758573217728711

ELBOW MANIPULATION TECHNIQUES

Humeral ulnar joint - seated

- The patient is seated on the table, while sitting firmly on the palmar aspect of the hand on the affected side to reinforce.

- Stand or sit next to the patient, and, using both hands, securely contact a pisiform–hypothenar contact on the anterior aspect of the humeral/ ulnar joint.

- The patient's weight on their hand stabilises the arm while the therapist performs the manipulation as shown.

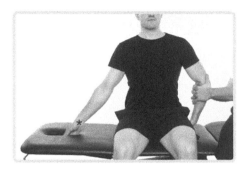

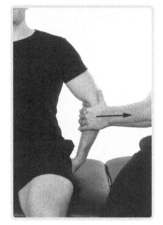

Radial head - seated with thumb contact

- Stand on the side of the arm to be manipulated.

- Stand with an asymmetrical stance.

- Supinate the elbow and locate and palpate the medial aspect of the radial head; using your thumb, apply that as a fulcrum behind the radial head, ensuring you take out the tissue slack.

- With your other hand, grasp around the inside of the patient's wrist and pronate.

- The movement is a 50/50 between your left and right hand; as you flex the elbow, you will add pronation to bring the radial head more lateral.

- Engage the barrier and perform the manipulation by applying a short thrust towards the glenohumeral joint.

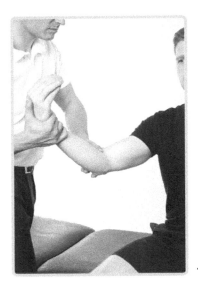

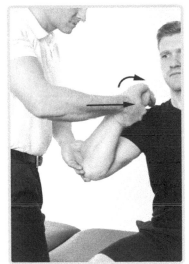

Radial head - seated with pisiform contact

- Stand on the side of the arm to be manipulated.

- Stand with an asymmetrical stance.

- Supinate the elbow and locate and palpate the medial aspect of the radial head; using your pisiform, apply that as a fulcrum behind the radial head, ensuring you take out the tissue slack.

- With your other hand, grasp around the inside of the patient's wrist and pronate.

- The movement is a 50/50 between your left and right hand; as you flex the elbow, you will add pronation to bring the radial head more lateral.

- Engage the barrier and perform the manipulation by applying a short thrust towards the glenohumeral joint.

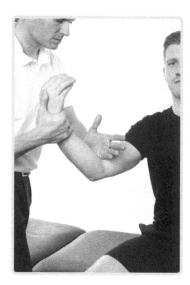

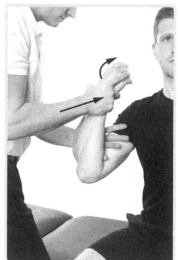

Radial head - seated with pisiform contact

- The technique can also be applied supine, seated or recumbent.

- Stand on the side of the arm to be manipulated.

- Stand with an asymmetrical stance.

- Locate and palpate the lateral aspect of the radial head.

- With your other hand, grasp around the patient's wrist and pronate the forearm to 45° (so their thumb is now facing downwards); get the patient to lean away from you, which will increase slight traction of the joint and help to take up the tissue tension.

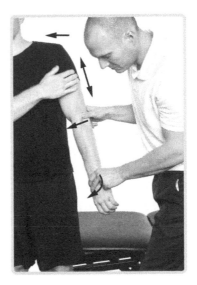

- Engage the barrier and perform the manipulation by pronating the forearm, flexing the wrist and fully extending the elbow while applying pressure to the radial head, moving it obliquely.

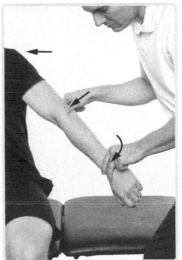

Prone radial head manipulation

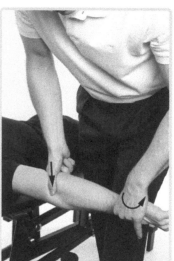

- The patient is prone.

- Stand on the side of the arm to be manipulated.

- Stand with an asymmetrical stance.

- Locate and palpate the lateral aspect of the radial head, and traction the elbow.

- With your other hand, grasp around the patient's wrist and pronate the forearm to 45° (so their thumb is now facing downwards).

- Engage the barrier and perform the manipulation by pronating the forearm, flexing the wrist and fully extending the elbow while applying pressure to the radial head, moving it obliquely.

Seated long-axis distraction of the humeroradial joint

- The patient should be seated.

- Stand on the side of the arm to be manipulated, with the elbow in slight flexion.

- Stand with an asymmetrical stance.

- Take hold of the distal forearm and with the contact hand use a web contact over the distal humerus.

- Add slight traction with the stabilising hand; the contact hand thrusts in an oblique angle to the humeroradial joint.

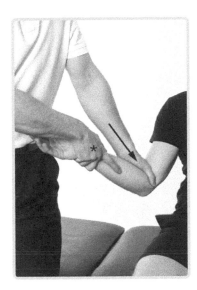

Long-axis radial head manipulation using a fulcrum

- The patient should be supine.

- Stand on the side of the arm to be manipulated; contacting the elbow, a fulcrum should be placed underneath the medial epicondyle, as shown.

- Stand with an asymmetrical stance, stabilising the shoulder on the affected side with one hand while contacting the elbow of the affected side with the other hand.

- Add slight pronation of the wrist to bring the radial head round.

- Start to increase the pressure on the shoulder and the wrist equally.

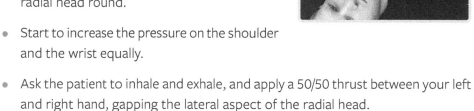

- Ask the patient to inhale and exhale, and apply a 50/50 thrust between your left and right hand, gapping the lateral aspect of the radial head.

Prone, posterior to anterior humeral ulnar joint

- The patient should be prone.

- Stand on the side of the arm to be manipulated.

- With the arm extended, the contact hand uses a thenar hypothenar contact over the olecranon.

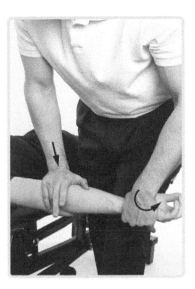

- Add slight pronation of the wrist to bring the palmar side facing upwards.

- Start to increase the pressure on the olecranon.

- Ask the patient to inhale and exhale, and apply a short impulse thrust, posterior to anterior.

Seated, posterior to anterior humeral ulnar joint

- The patient should be seated.

- Stand to the side of the target joint.

- Support the medial and lateral epicondyle of the humerus with a thenar hypothenar contact.

- Your other hand grasps around the patient's wrist.

- The manipulation is generated by your right hand extending the elbow via the wrist and simultaneously moving the dominant hand superiorly, pressing into the medial and lateral humeral condyles.

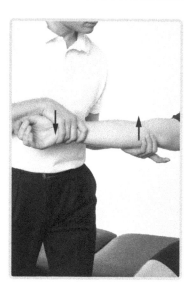

Supine, medial to lateral gapping of the humeroulnar joint

- The patient should be supine.

- Abduct the elbow to allow you to step into the space contacting the medial aspect of the elbow joint.

- Stand to the medial aspect of the target joint.

- Stabilise the patient's forearm against your body, using the outside hip to support the forearm.

- The contact hand is on the medial aspect of the elbow, with the thumb sitting over the joint line.

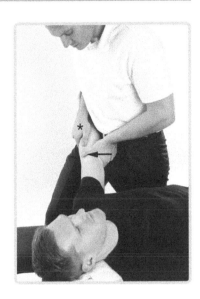

- Using your body to brace the elbow, you will stress the elbow medially to laterally.

- A short thrust is introduced at the medial aspect of the elbow to gap the lateral aspect.

Supine, lateral to medial gapping of the humeroulnar joint

- The patient should be supine.

- Abduct the elbow while standing on the lateral aspect.

- Stabilise the patient's forearm against your body, using the outside hip to support the forearm.

- The contact hand is on the lateral aspect of the elbow, with the thumb sitting over the joint line.

- Using your body to brace the elbow, stress the elbow lateral to medial.

- A short thrust is introduced at the lateral aspect of the elbow to gap the medial aspect.

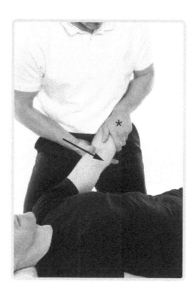

Seated, lateral to medial gapping of the humeroulnar joint

- The patient should be seated and leaning away.

- Abduct the elbow to allow you to step into the space contacting the medial aspect of the elbow joint.

- Stabilise the patient's forearm against your body, using the outside hip to support the forearm.

- The contact hand is on the medial aspect of the elbow, with the thumb sitting over the joint line.

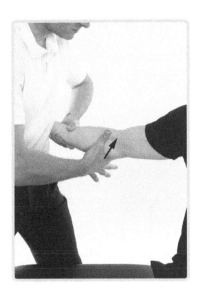

- Using your body to brace the elbow, stress the elbow medially to laterally.

- A short thrust is introduced at the medial aspect of the elbow to gap the lateral aspect.

Seated, lateral to medial gapping of the humeroulnar joint

- The patient should be seated.

- Abduct the elbow while standing on the lateral aspect.

- Stabilise the patient's forearm against your body, using the outside hip to support the forearm.

- The contact hand is on the lateral aspect of the elbow, with the thumb sitting over the joint line.

- Using your body to brace the elbow, stress the elbow lateral to medial.

- A short thrust is introduced at the lateral aspect of the elbow to gap the medially aspect.

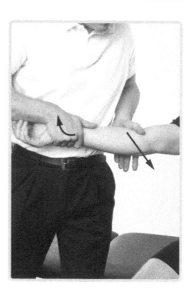

Prone, medial to lateral gapping of the humeroulnar joint

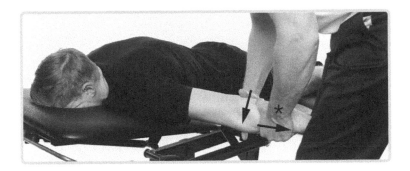

- The patient should be prone.

- Bring the patient's arm to 90° and, using your legs, stabilise the forearm between your legs just above the knees; this will allow you to lean back to traction the elbow joint.

- The contact hand is above the elbow on the medial aspect and the other hand is below the lateral aspect of the elbow, with the thumb sitting over the joint line.

- Using your body to traction back and the medial contact hand, stress the elbow joint, lateral to medial.

- A short thrust is introduced at the medial side to gap the lateral.

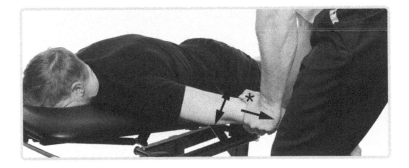

- Adaption: a bilateral contact below the elbow joint line allows you to stabilise the elbow. Using both hands, stress the elbow joint, performing a short thrust towards the lateral side.

Prone, lateral to medial gapping of the humeroulnar joint

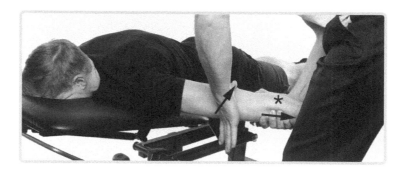

- The patient should be prone.

- Bring the patient's arm to 90° and, using your legs, stabilise the forearm between your legs just above the knees; this will allow you to lean back to traction the elbow joint.

- The contact hand is above the elbow on the lateral aspect and the other hand is below the medial aspect of the elbow, with the thumb sitting over the joint line.

- Using your body to traction back and the lateral contact hand, stress the elbow joint, lateral to medial.

- A short thrust is introduced at the lateral side to gap the medial side.

- Adaption: a bilateral contact below the elbow joint line allows you to stabilise the elbow. Using both hands, stress the elbow joint, performing a short thrust towards the medial side (see the picture above).

WRIST MANIPULATION TECHNIQUES

Thumb/1st MCP manipulation

- The patient is in a recumbent position with the therapist standing on the affected side.

- With your left hand, hold the patient's thumb as shown, using a pisiform contact over the joint.

- Your right hand stabilises and holds down the wrist.

- Your hand fixes down in the plateau between the 1st metacarpal joint and the trapezium.

- Use your hand to grip and traction the 1st metacarpal – this will open the joint space of the 1st metacarpal – then place your application (manipulating thumb, as shown) over the joint line.

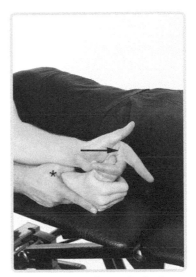

1st metacarpal manipulation

- Place your palmar surface over your other hand, reinforcing the posterior surface of your 1st metacarpal phalangeal joint.

- You can extend your arms slightly, creating extension and traction applied to the patient's proximal end of their 1st metacarpal joint.

- Ask the patient to inhale and exhale.

- As the patient exhales, engage the barrier. Apply a traction manipulation distracting the joint.

Carpal manipulation - inferior drive

- With the patient prone, take the wrist and traction backwards while you hold the patient's fully pronated hand with the contact hand, as shown.

- Locate the desired carpal bone to manipulate and contact your thumb over it; reinforce the thumb with the pisiform of the other hand.

- Flex and extend the patient's wrist with momentum.

- The manipulation is directed towards the palmar aspect of the hand as you move the wrist into extension.

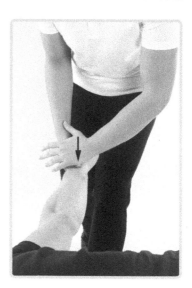

Carpal manipulation - superior drive

- With the patient prone, take the wrist and traction backwards while you hold the patient's fully supinated hand with the contact hand, as shown.

- Locate the desired carpal bone to manipulate and contact your thumb over it; reinforce the thumb with the pisiform of the other hand.

- Flex and extend the patient's wrist with momentum.

- The manipulation is directed towards the palmar aspect of the hand as you move the wrist into flexion.

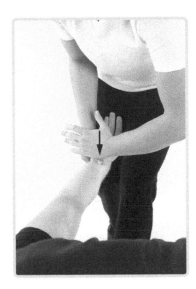

Distal ulnar

- The patient is in a recumbent position with the therapist standing on the affected side.

- With your left hand, hold the patient's distal ulnar over the joint.

- Your right hand stabilises and tractions the wrist away from the distal ulnar, creating space.

- Under traction bring the wrist up in a superior line with the right hand, while the left hand applies an inferior glide downwards with the left hand.

- Ask the patient to inhale and exhale.

- As the patient exhales, engage the barrier. The left and right hand create a shearing thrust, which is applied, distracting the joint.

Distal radius

- The patient is in a recumbent position, with the therapist standing on the affected side.

- With your left hand, hold the patient's distal radius over the joint.

- Your right hand stabilises and tractions the wrist away from the distal ulnar, creating space.

- Under traction bring the wrist down in an inferior line with the right hand, while the left hand applies a superior glide downwards with the left hand.

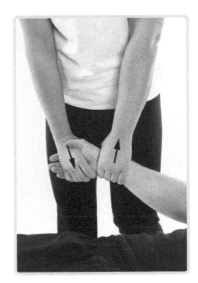

- Ask the patient to inhale and exhale.

- As the patient exhales, engage the barrier. The left hand and right hand create a shearing thrust, which is applied, distracting the joint.

8

THE LUMBAR SPINE

Introduction

Spinal manipulation is a treatment method regularly used by various healthcare professionals including osteopaths, chiropractors and physical therapists to treat problems of the lumbar spine (Dorron *et al.* 2016). Common therapeutic scenarios that involve the use of lumbar spine manipulation (LSM) include treatment for low back pain (LBP) and lumbar disc herniation (Hincapié *et al.* 2018; Shokri *et al.* 2018; Tudini *et al.* 2016). It is worth noting that LBP is estimated to affect 70–80 per cent of all individuals at some point in their lifetime, with an economic burden of over US$100 billion annually in the USA and over £12 billion in the UK (Allegri *et al.* 2016; Dagenais, Caro and Haldeman 2017; Dorron *et al.* 2016; Tudini *et al.*, 2016). While there are some clinicians with reservations about using LSM in the management of LBP (Hincapié *et al.* 2018), its utility cannot be ignored as various studies have shown positive benefits and very rare complications (<1 in 3.7 million) arising from the treatment (Olson 2016; Shokri *et al.* 2018). In its guidelines, the National Institute for Health and Care Excellence (NICE) (2016) recommends spinal manipulation along with other forms of manual therapy for managing LBP. As with many pathological conditions, the therapist needs to accurately diagnose the etiological factors contributing to LBP before performing LSM.

This chapter discusses the joints of the lumbar spine and their range of motion, common injuries, important red flags and appropriate special tests to help LSM therapists identify serious pathology in this section of the vertebral column.

Joints

The lumbar spine consists of five articulating vertebrae (L1–L5) (see Table 8.1) along with the associated muscles, ligaments and tendons (Bogduk and Bogduk 2012; Cooper 2015). This region of the spine is bordered by thoracic vertebrae cranially and sacral bones caudally. The lumbar vertebrae are distinctly large, lack costal facets and transverse foramina (Standring 2016; Waxenbaum and Futterman 2018). In the lumbar region, the ten zygapophysial joints lie in the sagittal plane, with the articulating facets at angles of 90° and 45° respectively to the transverse and coronal planes (Hamill, Knutzen and Derrick 2014). Superior facets face the median while the inferior facets are oriented laterally with a change occurring at the lumbosacral junction, where the facet joint 'moves into the frontal plane and the inferior facet on L5 faces front' (Hamill *et al.* 2014, p.251). The orientational adjustment at the lumbosacral junction prevents the vertebral column from gliding frontward on the sacrum (Hamill *et al.* 2014). Lumbar vertebrae articulate to provide for motion while concomitantly bearing the weight of the spine and protecting neural tissue (Cooper 2015).

Table 8.1. Joints of the lumbar spine

Joint name	Description	Function
Symphyseal joints (secondary cartilaginous joints)	• Articulations between the bodies of adjacent vertebrae	• Allow slight movement between the vertebrae • Provide support during high-impact activities and load bearing
Zygapophysial joints (apophyseal joints, facet joints)	• Synovial joints formed from articulation of the vertebral articular processes of neighbouring vertebrae	• Restrict anterior translation and flexion of the vertebral segment • Provide for gliding and gapping motion • Facilitate rotation
Fibrous joints	• These articulations result from the direct connection of adjacent vertebrae by fibrous connective tissue • They join the laminae, transverse and spinous processes of lumbar vertebrae	• Stabilise the vertebral column in position

Sources: Bogduk and Bogduk (2012); Olson (2016); OpenStax (2018); Standring (2016); Watson, Paxinos and Kayalioglu (2009)

Range of motion

Articulations of the lumbar spine provide for axial compression, axial distraction, flexion, extension, axial rotation and lateral flexion (Bogduk and Bogduk 2012; Cooper 2015) (see Table 8.2). Studies have reported the active range of motion of the lumbar spine as 52–60° flexion, 15–37° extension, 14–26° lateral flexion (left and right) and 30° rotation (left and right) (Hamill *et al.* 2014; Olson 2016). It is important to note that movements at the lumbar spine are difficult to measure clinically, because of significant variation among people. A number of reasons also affect the measuring of the range of motion such as age, sex, genetic make-up, pathological condition and laxity of ligaments (McKenzie and May 2003) (see Table 8.3).

Table 8.2. Maximal and minimal median ranges of lumbar spinal motion across various subjects with an overall age range of 16–90

Movement	Male		Female	
	Maximum (median of values)	Minimum	Maximum (median of values)	Minimum
Flexion	73°	40°	68°	40°
Extension	29°	7°	28°	6°
Right lateral flexion	28°	15°	27°	14°
Left lateral flexion	28°	16°	28°	18°
Right axial rotation	7°	7°	8°	8°
Left axial rotation	7°	7°	6°	6°

Source: Troke et al. (2005)

Table 8.3. Ranges of segmental motion for the lumbar spine in males aged between 25 and 36

Mean range (Measured in degrees, with standard deviations)							
Level	Flexion (forward bending)	Extension (backward bending)	Flexion and extension	Lateral flexion		Axial rotation	
				Left	Right	Left	Right
L1–L2	8° (5°)	5° (2°)	13° (5°)	5°	6°	1°	1°
L2–L3	10° (2°)	3° (2°)	13° (2°)	5°	6°	1°	1°
L3–L4	12° (1°)	1° (1°)	13° (2°)	5°	6°	1°	2°
L4–L5	13° (4°)	2° (1°)	16° (4°)	3°	5°	1°	2°
L5–S1	9° (6°)	5° (4°)	14° (5°)	0	2°	1°	0

Source: Adapted from Bogduk and Bogduk (2012); see also Pearcy and Tibrewal (1984); Pearcy, Portek and Shepherd (1984)

Common injuries

The lumbar spine often suffers injuries resulting from various events such as motor vehicle accidents, sporting accidents or other external forces beyond the strength of the vertebrae. The intensity of the injuries varies on a continuum from mild to severe, with the latter category including various types of fracture, spondylolysis, spondylolistheses and disc herniations among others (Dunn, Proctor and Day 2006) (see Table 8.4).

Table 8.4. Common injuries of the lumbar spine

Common injuries	Characteristics
Soft-tissue injuries	• Muscle sprains (ligament damage) and strains (injury to muscle or tendon) • Local tenderness with no radiculopathy • Symptoms are aggravated by heavy continuous exercise of the spinal muscles
Lumbar disc herniation	• Frequently the result of wear and tear of the intervertebral discs • Frequency is higher in people exposed to considerable axial loading, rotation and flexion such as athletes, although also frequent in adults • Indications include numbness of legs sometimes accompanied by loss of leg function, dull or sharp pain, sciatica, muscle spasm or cramping, and weakness
Spondylolysis and spondylolisthesis	• Usually occurs at L5 (L5–S1) resulting from activities involving recurring hyperextension and axial loading • LBP with no radiculopathy • Symptoms may be intensified by extension • Common in active young people
Compression fracture	• Causes the anterior part of the vertebra to break and lose height • Rarely leads to neurological problems • Frequent in osteoporosis patients
Vertebral body fracture	• Linked with high-impact accidents and osteoporosis • Often leads to development of neural deficits that include a feeling of numbness, faintness, tingling, spinal and neurogenic shock • Higher frequency in men than women

Sources: Dunn et al. *(2006); Ombregt (2013)*

Red flags

Red flags are features of history taking that are useful in identifying significant pathology in patients suffering from lumbar pain (McKenzie and May 2003; Verhagen *et al.* 2016) (see Table 8.5). Verhagen *et al.* (2017) indicate that it is unclear which red flags are relevant, citing a lack of empirical support for many red flags in the diagnosis of LBP. If red flag pathology is suspected in a patient, the therapist should use sound clinical reasoning to reduce the patient's risk of adverse events following LSM.

Table 8.5. Red flags for serious pathology in the lumbar spine

Condition	Incidence (estimated)	Signs and symptoms
Cauda equine syndrome	Ranges from 1 in 33,000 to 1 in 100,000	• Urinary or faecal incontinence • Bowel incontinence or lack of control over defecation • Saddle anaesthesia (perianal/perineal) or paraesthesia • Global or progressive motor weakness in lower extremities • Sensory deficiencies in the feet (L4, L5 and S1 areas) • Ankle dorsiflexion, toe extension, as well as ankle plantar flexion weakness
Malignancy	Prevalence between 0.1% and 3.5%	• Age >50 years • History of cancer • Unintentional or unexplained weight loss • General malaise • Paraparesis • Persistent, progressive back 'pain at night' or 'pain at rest'
Possible infection	1 per 250,000 of the general population	• Fever (≥38°C) or chills • Recent infection (urinary tract or skin) • Immunodeficiency/AIDS • Penetrating wound near spine • Pain (intense night pain or pain at rest, or bone tenderness over the lumbar spinous process) • Intravenous drug use or abuse • Concurrent immunosuppressive disorder • No recovery after six weeks of conventional treatment
Spinal fracture	Prevalence approximately 4%	• Age >50 years • History of trauma (past fractures as well as minor falls or heavy lifts for the elderly and patients with osteoporosis) • Protracted use of steroids • Pain (sudden severe onset, loading pain) • Structural deformity • Low bodyweight

Sources: Gardner, Gardner and Morley (2011); McKenzie and May (2003); Olson (2016); Verhagen et al. (2016)

Special tests

Therapists often use special tests to detect spinal instability in the lumbar region. These are clinically valid for the detection of the common pathologies associated with LBP, although thorough research is insufficient to ascertain this (Ferrari *et al.* 2015). This section presents a summary of some of the most common tests, associated positive signs and interpretations, shown in Table 8.6. It would be difficult to outline all the possible tests in this short chapter, so readers are encouraged to go through reference texts such as Olson's *Manual Physical Therapy of the Spine* (2016).

Table 8.6 is not an exhaustive list of special tests but gives you, the therapist, a guide for this area. If you are unsure of the interpretation of any test that you complete with your patient, we advise that you refer to the most appropriate medical professional for further investigations.

Table 8.6. Special tests for lumbar spine dysfunction

Test	Procedure	Positive sign	Interpretation
Straight leg raise Sensitivity = 0.80–0.97 Specificity = 0.4	The patient assumes a supine position on the treatment table with the therapist standing on the side to be examined. The therapist slowly flexes the patient's hip while maintaining the knee in full extension. The therapist should continually check for the patient's response and record the degree of hip flexion attained when symptoms are reported. The procedure is repeated with the other leg. Passive neck flexion may be added to increase dural tension	• Reduced angle of hip flexion (30° or less) and shooting pain proceeding from the lower back down to the posterior aspect of the thigh • Lower leg pain	✓ Nerve root irritation ✓ Herniated disc
Kemp's test Sensitivity = 0.35 Specificity = 0.47	The patient stands before the therapist, extending the spine as far as possible. Stabilising the ilium with one hand while grabbing the shoulder with the other hand, the therapist applies overpressure, gently leading the patient to extension with the patient laterally flexing and rotating to the side of pain. The therapist sustains this position for approximately 3 seconds	• Pain, numbness or stinging in the area of the back or lower limb	✓ Localised pain suggests facet syndrome ✓ Radiating pain toward the leg is indicative of nerve root irritation

Test	Procedure	Positive sign	Interpretation
Slump test Specificity = 0.83 Sensitivity = 0.84	The patient sits erect on the edge of the treatment table, with the posterior knee crease at the edge of the side or foot of the table. Symptoms are noted before the patient is asked to slump, collapsing the thoracic and lumbar spines into flexion while the head and neck are kept from flexing. Gentle overpressure is applied to the upper thoracic area. The patient is then instructed to fully flex the neck, bringing the chin to the sternum, and the therapist applies gentle overpressure to the flexed spine. While maintaining the overpressure, the patient is instructed to extend one knee as far as possible and at the same time the therapist dorsiflexes the ankle. The patient narrates what they are feeling to the therapist at each step during the procedure	• Reproduction of radicular pain in the back or lower limb	✓ Increased sciatic nerve root tension

Sources: Kamath and Kamath (2017); Majlesi et al. (2008); Olson (2016); Stuber et al. (2014); Wise (2015)

The lumbar spine is both robust and delicate, withstanding a great amount of biomechanical forces, while at the same time it is not immune to pathologies such as LBP and others. When the population is affected by LBP, this has a telling effect on the economy of a nation, and effective treatment modalities would be imperative. As therapists study the intricate anatomy of the lumbar region, the biomechanics thereof and common pathological conditions affecting it, they will become more comfortable with therapeutic interventions such as LSM. It is necessary, however, for the therapist to carefully assess cases on an individual basis before deciding to treat with LSM or any other treatment method.

References

Allegri, M., Montella, S., Salici, F., Valente, A., Marchesini, M., Compagnone, C. *et al.* (2016) 'Mechanisms of low back pain: A guide for diagnosis and therapy.' *F1000Research 5*, 1530. doi:10.12688/f1000research.8105.2

Bogduk, N. and Bogduk, N. (2012) *Clinical and Radiological Anatomy of the Lumbar Spine.* Amsterdam: Elsevier/Churchill Livingstone.

Cooper, G. (2015) *Non-Operative Treatment of the Lumbar Spine.* Cham: Springer International Publishing. doi:10.1007/978-3-319-21443-6

Dagenais, S., Caro, J. and Haldeman, S. (2017) 'A systematic review of low back pain cost of illness studies in the United States and internationally.' *The Spine Journal 8*(1), 8–20. doi:10.1016/j.spinee.2007.10.005

Dorron, S.L., Losco, B.E., Drummond, P.D. and Walker, B.F. (2016) 'Effect of lumbar spinal manipulation on local and remote pressure pain threshold and pinprick sensitivity in asymptomatic individuals: A randomised trial.' *Chiropractic & Manual Therapies 24*(1), 47. doi:10.1186/s12998-016-0128-5

Dunn, I.F., Proctor, M.R. and Day, A.L. (2006) 'Lumbar spine injuries in athletes.' *Neurosurgical Focus 21*(4), E4. doi:10.1016/B978-0-323-06952-6.00070-1

Ferrari, S., Manni, T., Bonetti, F., Villafañe, J.H. and Vanti, C. (2015) 'A literature review of clinical tests for lumbar instability in low back pain: Validity and applicability in clinical practice.' *Chiropractic & Manual Therapies 23*, 14. doi:10.1186/s12998-015-0058-7

Gardner, A., Gardner, E. and Morley, T. (2011) 'Cauda equina syndrome: A review of the current clinical and medico-legal position.' *European Spine Journal 20*(5), 690–697. doi:10.1007/s00586-010-1668-3

Hamill, J., Knutzen, K. and Derrick, T.R. (2014) *Biomechanical Basis of Human Movement*. Philadelphia, PA: Wolters Kluwer.

Hincapié, C.A., Cassidy, J.D., Côté, P., Rampersaud, Y.R., Jadad, A.R. and Tomlinson, G.A. (2018) 'Chiropractic spinal manipulation and the risk for acute lumbar disc herniation: A belief elicitation study.' *European Spine Journal 27*(7), 1517–1525. doi:10.1007/s00586-017-5295-0

Kamath, S.U. and Kamath, S.S. (2017) 'Lasègue's sign.' *Journal of Clinical and Diagnostic Research 11*(5), RG01–RG02. doi:10.7860/JCDR/2017/24899.9794

Majlesi, J., Togay, H., Unalan, H. and Toprak, S. (2008) 'The sensitivity and specificity of the slump and the straight leg raising tests in patients with lumbar disc herniation.' *Journal of Clinical Rheumatology 14*(2), 87–91. doi:10.1097/RHU.0b013e31816b2f99

McKenzie, R. and May, S. (2003) *The Lumbar Spine: Mechanical Diagnosis and Therapy*. Volume 1. Waikanae, New Zealand: Spinal Publications New Zealand.

NICE (National Institute for Health and Care Excellence) (2016) 'Low back pain and sciatica in over 16s: Assessment and management.' NICE guideline. Available at www.nice.org.uk/guidance/ng59/resources/low-back-pain-and-sciatica-in-over-16s-assessment-and-management-pdf-1837521693637

Olson, K.A. (2016) *Manual Physical Therapy of the Spine*. 2nd edn. St Louis, MO: Elsevier.

Ombregt, L. (2013) *A System of Orthopaedic Medicine*. London: Churchill Livingstone.

OpenStax (2018) *Anatomy and Physiology*. OpenStax College. Available at https://openstax.org/details/books/anatomy-and-physiology

Pearcy, M.J. and Tibrewal, S.B. (1984) 'Axial rotation and lateral bending in the normal lumbar spine measured by three-dimensional radiography.' *Spine 9*(6), 582–587. Available at www.ncbi.nlm.nih.gov/pubmed/6495028

Pearcy, M., Portek, I. and Shepherd, J. (1984) 'Three-dimensional x-ray analysis of normal movement in the lumbar spine.' *Spine 9*(3), 294–297. Available at www.ncbi.nlm.nih.gov/pubmed/6374922

Shokri, E., Kamali, F., Sinaei, E. and Ghafarinejad, F. (2018) 'Spinal manipulation in the treatment of patients with MRI-confirmed lumbar disc herniation and sacroiliac joint hypomobility: A quasi-experimental study.' *Chiropractic & Manual Therapies 26*(1), 16. doi:10.1186/s12998-018-0185-z

Standring, S. (ed.) (2016) *Gray's Anatomy: The Anatomical Basis of Clinical Practice*. 41st edn. New York: Elsevier. Available at www.elsevier.com/books/grays-anatomy/standring/978-0-7020-5230-9

Stuber, K., Lerede, C., Kristmanson, K., Sajko, S. and Bruno, P. (2014) 'The diagnostic accuracy of the Kemp's test: A systematic review.' *The Journal of the Canadian Chiropractic Association 58*(3), 258–267. Available at www.ncbi.nlm.nih.gov/pubmed/25202153

Troke, M., Moore, A.P., Maillardet, F.J. and Cheek, E. (2005) 'A normative database of lumbar spine ranges of motion.' *Manual Therapy 10*(3), 198–206. doi:10.1016/j.math.2004.10.004

Tudini, F., Chui, K., Grimes, J., Laufer, R., Kim, S., Yen, S.-C. *et al.* (2016) 'Cervical spine manual therapy for aging and older adults.' *Topics in Geriatric Rehabilitation 32*(2), 88–105. doi:10.1097/TGR.0000000000000075

Verhagen, A.P., Downie, A., Maher, C. and Koes, B.W. (2017) 'Most red flags for malignancy in low back pain guidelines lack empirical support: A systematic review.' *Pain.* doi:10.1097/j. pain.0000000000000998

Verhagen, A.P., Downie, A., Popal, N., Maher, C. and Koes, B.W. (2016) 'Red flags presented in current low back pain guidelines: A review.' *European Spine Journal 25*(9), 2788–2802. doi:10.1007/s00586-016-4684-0

Watson, C., Paxinos, G. and Kayalioglu, G. (eds) (2009) *The Spinal Cord: A Christopher and Dana Reeve Foundation Text and Atlas.* Amsterdam: Elsevier/Academic Press.

Waxenbaum, J.A. and Futterman, B. (2018) 'Anatomy, Back, Lumbar Vertebrae.' *StatPearls.* Available at www.ncbi.nlm.nih.gov/pubmed/29083618

Wise, C.H. (2015) *Orthopaedic Manual Physical Therapy: From Art to Evidence.* Philadelphia, PA: F.A. Davis Company.

LUMBAR SPINE MANIPULATION TECHNIQUES

Lumbar spine manipulation with rotation, L1-L5/S1

- Ask the patient to lie on their side. Their body should be in a straight line.

- The head is in a neutral position, supported using a pillow.

- The spine is straight, with no rotation. The bottom leg on the table is straight, the top leg bent with a 90° position at the hip (if possible) and the foot rests in the popliteal crease of the bottom knee. The patient should have their arms in a folded position in front of their chest.

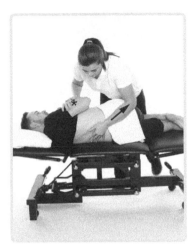

- Stand at the side of the table facing the patient. This is a wide split stance with slight rotation of the front/lead leg forward towards the patient's head, the inner part of your leg contacting the table. Your back leg is behind, approximately at the patient's hip level, with the outer aspect of the leg in contact with the table.

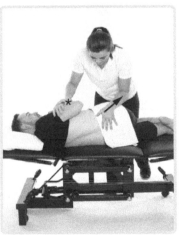

- Holding the patient's lower arm, rotate the body until you reach the desired segment.

- Once set-up is complete to the desired segment, rotate the patient's body towards you.

- The contact of your hand should be over the target segment spinous processes (SPs) or posterior superior iliac spine (PSIS) with an angle towards the femur as this will be your line of drive.

- Ask the patient to breathe in and out. As they start the out breath, begin to engage the barrier by rotating the upper body away from you with your hand and rotating the lumbar.

- As you reach the barrier, your impulse for the manipulation is down the line of the femur, gained by dropping your bodyweight down the line of the femur of the affected side.

Key to note:

- When performing the set-up, you know you are at the desired level when the target SP begins to rotate and pushes against your palpating hand, which we call 'standing proud'.

- Getting the lumbar SPs to face the ceiling allows you the correct leverage point for the lumbar spine (LSP) and means you use less force and more bodyweight, which makes it easier for you.

- Remember your applicator can be your fingers, flat palm, ulnar border or extensors/flexors of the forearm (which we prefer, as this is the balance of comfort for them and joint safety for you).

- When using a thigh contact, use a towel to create a barrier for the patient.

- Remember not to keep the patient at the barrier for too long.

- Always help the patient back to the supine position.

Lumbar spine body drop manipulation with rotation, L1-L5/S1

- Ask the patient to lie on their side. Their body should be in a straight line.

- The head is in a neutral position, supported using a pillow.

- The spine is straight, with no rotation. The bottom leg on the table is straight, the top leg bent with a 90° position at the hip (if possible), and the foot rests in the popliteal crease of the bottom knee. The patient should have their arms in a folded position in front of their chest.

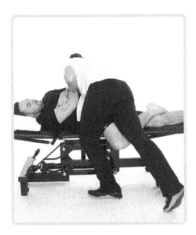

- Stand at the side of the table, facing the patient. This is a wide split stance with slight rotation of the front/lead leg forward towards the patient's head, the inner part of your leg contacting the table. Your back leg is behind, approximately at the patient's hip level, with the outer aspect of the leg in contact with the table.

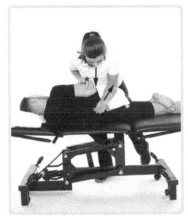

- Holding the patient's lower arm, rotate the body until you reach the desired segment.

- Once set-up is complete to the desired segment, rotate the patient's body towards you so that the SPs of the lumbar spine are almost facing the ceiling.

- The contact of your hand should be over the PSIS with an angle towards the femur, as this will be your line of drive.

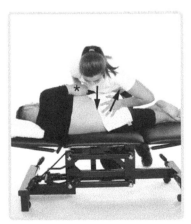

- Your thigh will then contact the thigh of the patient.

- Ask the patient to breathe in and out. As they start the out breath, begin to engage the barrier by rotating the upper body away from you with your hand and rotating the lumbar spine towards you.

- Rotate the lumbar spine towards you via your contact over the PSIS and your thigh contact.

- As you reach the barrier, your impulse for the manipulation is down the line of the femur, gained by dropping your upper body through your rotating arm contact aided by the downward movement of your thigh – all down the line of the femur of the affected side.

Key to note:

- When performing the set-up, you know that you are at the desired level when the target SP begins to rotate and pushes against your palpating hand, which we call 'standing proud'.

- Getting the lumbar SPs to face the ceiling allows you the correct leverage point for the LSP and means you use less force and more bodyweight, which makes it easier for you.

- Remember your applicator can be your fingers, flat palm, ulnar border or extensors/flexors of the forearm (which we prefer, as this is the balance of comfort for them and joint safety for you).

- When using a thigh contact, use a towel to create a barrier for the patient.

- Remember not to keep the patient at the barrier for too long.

- Always help the patient back to the supine position.

Lumbar spine PSIS contact no rotation, L1-L5/S1

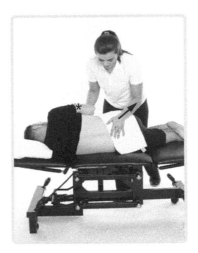

- Ask the patient to lie on their side on the table. Their body should be in a straight line.

- The head is in a neutral position, supported using a pillow or towel.

- The spine is straight, with no rotation. The bottom leg on the table is straight, the top leg bent with a 90° position at the hip (if possible), and the foot rests in the popliteal crease of the bottom knee. The patient should have their arms in a folded position in front of their chest.

- Stand at the side of the table facing the patient. This is a wide split stance with slight rotation of the front/lead leg forward towards the patient's head, the inner part of your leg contacting the table. Your back leg is behind, approximately at the patient's hip level, with the outer aspect of the leg in contact with the table.

- Once set-up is complete to the desired segment, rotate the patient's body towards you so that the SPs of the lumbar spine are almost facing the ceiling.

- The contact of your hand should be over the PSIS with an angle towards the femur, as this will be your line of drive.

- Ask the patient to breathe in and out. As they start the out breath, begin to engage the barrier by rotating the upper body away from you with your hand and rotating the lumbar spine towards you.

- Rotate the lumbar spine towards you via your contact over the PSIS.

- As you reach the barrier, your impulse for the manipulation is down the line of the femur via the PSIS of the affected side.

Key to note:

- This technique helps when the patient is much heavier then you or is unable to complete the normal rotation for a variety of different reasons but is safe to treat.

- Getting the lumbar SPs to face the ceiling allows you the correct leverage point for the LSP and means you use less force and more bodyweight, which makes it easier for you.

- Remember your applicator can be your fingers, flat palm, ulnar border or extensors/flexors of the forearm (which we prefer, as this is the balance of comfort for them and joint safety for you).

- Use a towel to create a barrier for the patient for your hand on the forearms and over the PSIS.

- Remember not to keep the patient at the barrier for too long.

- Always help the patient back to the supine position if it is easier for them.

Lumbar spine thenar contact on specific segment or PSIS no rotation, L1-L5/S1

- Ask the patient to lie on their side on the table. Their body should be in a straight line.

- The head is in a neutral position, supported using a pillow or towel.

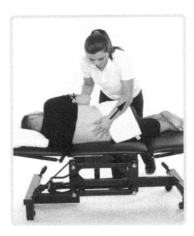

- The spine is straight, with no rotation. The bottom leg on the table is straight, the top leg bent with a 90° position at the hip (if possible), and the foot rests in the popliteal crease of the bottom knee. The patient should have their arms in a folded position in front of their chest.

- Stand at the side of the table facing the patient. This is a wide split stance with slight rotation of the front/lead leg forward towards the patient's head, the inner part of your leg contacting the table. Your back leg is behind, approximately at the patient's hip level, with the outer aspect of the leg in contact with the table.

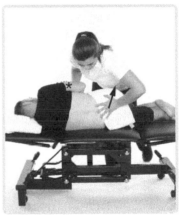

- Once set-up is complete to the desired segment, rotate the patient's body towards you via the specific SP or PSIS so that the SPs of the lumbar spine are almost facing the ceiling.

- The contact of your hand should be over the specific segment you wish to manipulate or the PSIS with an angle towards you or the femur, as this will be your line of drive.

- Ask the patient to breathe in and out. As they start the out breath, begin to engage the barrier by rotating the upper body away from you with your hand and rotating the lumbar spine towards you.

- Rotate the lumbar spine towards you via your contact over the PSIS.

- As you reach the barrier, your impulse for the manipulation is in rotation at the specific segment or down the line of the femur via the PSIS of the affected side.

Key to note:

- This technique helps when the patient is much heavier then you or is unable to complete the normal rotation for a variety of different reasons but is safe to treat.

- There is no rotation in the set-up but there is during the manipulation that is created by you.

- Getting the lumbar SPs to face the ceiling allows you the correct leverage point for the LSP and means you use less force and more bodyweight, which makes it easier for you.

- Remember your applicator can be your fingers, flat palm, ulnar border or extensors/flexors of the forearm (which we prefer, as this is the balance of comfort for them and joint safety for you).

- Use a towel to create a barrier for the patient for your hand on the forearms and over the PSIS.

- Remember not to keep the patient at the barrier for too long.

- Always help the patient back to the supine position if it is easier for them.

Lumbar spine recumbent kick start with or without rotation, L1-L5/S1

- Ask the patient to lie on their side. Their body should be in a straight line.

- The head is in a neutral position, supported using a pillow.

- The spine is straight, with no rotation. The bottom leg on the table is straight, the top leg bent with a 90° position at the hip (if possible), and the foot rests in the popliteal crease of the bottom knee. The patient should have their arms in a folded position in front of their chest.

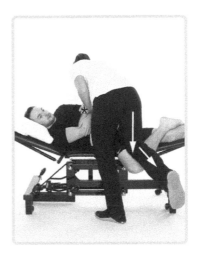

- Stand at the side of the table facing the patient.

- Incline the table to approximately 30° as this will help focus the set-up to your desired segment.

- This is a wide split stance with slight rotation of the front/lead leg forward towards the patient's head, the inner part of your leg contacting the table. Your back leg is behind, approximately at the patient's hip level, with the outer aspect of the leg in contact with the table.

- Holding the patient's lower arm, rotate the body until you reach the desired segment.

- Once set-up is complete to the desired segment, rotate the patient's body towards you so that the SPs of the lumbar spine are almost facing the ceiling.

- The contact of your hand should be over the PSIS with an angle towards the femur, as this will be your line of drive.

- Your knee will contact the popliteal groove angled with bias down the line of the femur.

- Ask the patient to breathe in and out. As they start the out breath, begin to engage the barrier by rotating the upper body away from you with your hand and rotating the lumbar spine towards you.

- Rotate the lumbar spine towards you via your contact over the PSIS and your thigh contact.

- As you reach the barrier, your impulse for the manipulation is down the line of the femur, gained by dropping your weight through your rotating arm contact aided by the downward movement of your leg via your knee – all down the line of the femur of the affected side.

Key to note:

- When performing the set-up, you know that you are at the desired level when the target SP begins to rotate and pushes against your palpating hand, which we call 'standing proud'.

- You can perform this manipulation without rotation of the upper body, if needed.

- Getting the lumbar SPs to face the ceiling allows you the correct leverage point for the LSP and means you use less force and more bodyweight, which makes it easier for you.

- Remember your applicator can be your fingers, flat palm, ulnar border or extensors/flexors of the forearm (which we prefer, as this is the balance of comfort for them and joint safety for you).

- When using a thigh contact, use a towel to create a barrier for the patient.

- Remember not to keep the patient at the barrier for too long.

- Always help the patient back to the supine position.

Lumbar spine manipulation modified with or without rotation and hip flexion, L1-L5/S1

- Ask the patient to lie on their side. Their body should be in a straight line.

- The head is in a neutral position, supported using a pillow.

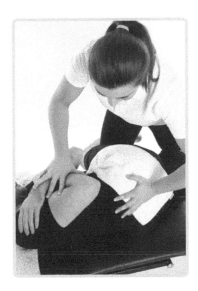

- The spine is straight, with no rotation. The bottom leg on the table is straight, the top leg bent with a 90° position at the hip (if possible), and the foot rests in the popliteal crease of the bottom knee. The patient should have their arms in a folded position in front of their chest.

- Stand at the side of the table, facing the patient. This is a wide split stance with slight rotation of the front/lead leg forward towards the patient's head, the inner part of your leg contacting the table. Your back leg is behind, approximately at the patient's hip level, with the outer aspect of the leg in contact with the table.

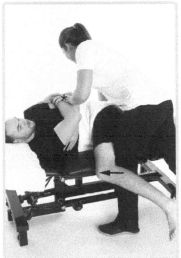

- Holding the patient's lower arm, rotate the body until you reached the desired segment.

- Once set-up is complete to the desired segment, rotate the patient's body towards you and, as you do this, allow the top leg to come off the table.

- Now step inside the top leg, as shown, making contact on the patient's popliteal crease or the hamstring if the patient is taller than you.

- The contact of your hand should be over the target segment SPs or PSIS with an angle towards the femur, as this will be your line of drive.

- Ask the patient to breathe in and out. As they start the out breath, begin to engage the barrier by rotating the upper body away from you with your hand and rotating the lumbar spine towards you while adding hip flexion with your leg contact.

- As you reach the barrier, your impulse for the manipulation is down the line of the femur, gained by dropping your bodyweight down the line of the femur of the affected side.

Key to note:

- When performing the set-up, you know that you are at the desired level when the target SP begins to rotate and pushes against your palpating hand, which we call 'standing proud'.

- The inclusion of hip flexion allows another vector and can be useful in both hyper- and hypomobile patients.

- Getting the lumbar SPs to face the ceiling allows you the correct leverage point for the LSP and means you use less force and more bodyweight, which makes it easier for you.

- Remember your applicator can be your fingers, flat palm, ulnar border or extensors/flexors of the forearm (which we prefer, as this is the balance of comfort for them and joint safety for you).

- When using a thigh contact, use a towel to create a barrier for the patient.

- Remember not to keep the patient at the barrier for too long.

- Always help the patient back to the supine position.

Lumbar spine manipulation seated, L1-L5/S1

- Ask the patient to be seated with folded arms or in the 'V' hold.

- Stand behind the patient at the side with an asymmetrical stance and gain contact on their elbows.

- The contact of your hand should be on the ipsilateral side of the target SP.

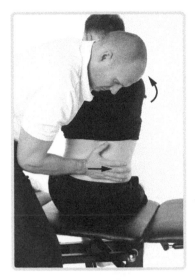

- Ask the patient to breathe in and out. As they start the out breath, begin to engage the barrier by rotating the upper body towards you while rotating the lumbar spine away from you via your contact, as shown.

- As you reach the barrier, your impulse for the manipulation is rotation of the upper body while aiding rotation of the target segment with your desired contact.

Key to note:

- The 'V' hold can be seen in the thoracic spine section if needed (use a towel for a barrier).

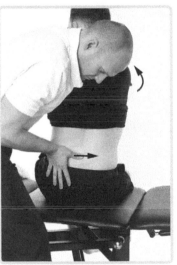

- When performing the set-up, you know that you are at the desired level when the target SP begins to rotate away from your palpating contact.

- Remember not to keep the patient at the barrier for too long.

9

PELVIS, HIP AND SACRUM

Introduction

Manipulative techniques are commonly used to treat lower back, hip, pelvic and buttock pain that originates from the lower body, particularly the pelvis and the sacroiliac joint (SIJ) (Gibbons and Tehan 2006; Laslett 2008). Various forms of manual medicine manipulation (e.g., manual therapy, osteopathic manual treatment, chiropractic adjustments) have been employed to yield substantial relief of pelvic and SIJ pain (Cohen, Chen and Neufeld 2013). This was demonstrated by a recent study that reported the efficacy of manipulation in treating a patient with SIJ dysfunction (Goldflies, Rosen and Hauser 2018). Another study found that high-velocity, low-amplitude (HVLA) SIJ manipulation, when combined with lumbar manipulation, yields positive results in patient treatment (Kamali and Shokri 2012). The latter results, in addition to demonstrating the efficacy of manipulation, illustrate the potential of hybrid approaches for manipulative treatment of the pelvis and SIJ.

The therapeutic goal of manual therapists in utilising manipulative techniques for pain relief in patients with pelvic and SIJ dysfunction is to provide a non-invasive, well-tolerated procedure that produces the best results. The ability of a therapist to comprehend the anatomy and physiology of the pelvic region and its associated joints will have a significant effect on patient outcomes (Ernst 2007; Gibbons and Tehan 2006; WHO 2005). Quite often, the knowledge and skills of the therapist have more to do with the actual outcome, for the patient, of any treatment. This chapter aims to provide therapists and associated professionals with brief descriptions of the joints of the pelvis, hip and sacrum, their ranges of motion and special diagnostic tests for detecting serious pathology. Later sections give an overview of common injuries to these structures and red flags to be aware of. The approach taken aims to aid development of knowledge for the target audience, with information that is both succinct and actionable.

Joints

The pelvis or the pelvic girdle comprises of paired coxal bones, the sacrum and the coccyx, and is interposed between the lower spinal column and the lower extremities (OpenStax 2018; Standring 2016). Each coxal bone is made up of three fused bones, namely, the ilium, ischium and pubis, and it is firmly attached to the axial skeleton at its articulation with the sacrum, at the SIJ (Standring 2016). The fused bones of the pelvis are immobile, providing a load-bearing scaffold to sustain the weight of the body. This provides stability, enabling the upper body to rest on the mobile limbs. Table 9.1 summarises the key joints located in the pelvic region.

Table 9.1. Joints of the pelvis and sacrum

Joint name	Description	Function
Acetabulofemoral joint	<ul><li>Commonly known as the 'hip joint'</li><li>A synovial, ball-and-socket joint</li><li>Found between the head of the femur with the acetabulum of the hip bone</li><li>Forms a connection between the lower limb and the pelvic girdle</li><li>Serves as a connection of the lower extremity with the axial skeleton of the trunk and pelvis</li></ul>	<ul><li>Facilitates bodyweight bearing in both dynamic and static postures</li><li>Maintains balance of the body</li></ul>
Sacroiliac joint	<ul><li>A matchless diarthrodial joint made up of the sacrum and the ilia of the pelvis</li><li>Forms a connection between the spine and the pelvis (ilium bones)</li><li>Usually formed within the sacral segments of S1, S2 and S3</li><li>Consists of fibrocartilage in addition to hyaline cartilage</li><li>Is a less mobile, well-innervated joint; thus, very strong and stable</li></ul>	<ul><li>Functions as a shock absorber for the spine</li><li>Conveys the weight of the upper extremity to the pelvis and legs</li><li>Offers steadiness to the spine and pelvis</li><li>Facilitates in the maintenance of body balance during walking (push-off phase)</li></ul>
Lumbosacral joint	<ul><li>A cartilaginous, multifunctional joint that connects the lumbar spine with the sacrum</li><li>Provides articulation between the vertebral bodies of the last lumbar vertebra (L5) and the first sacral segment (S1)</li><li>Consists of several interconnected components, including a disc between the two articulating vertebral bodies and two facet joints</li></ul>	<ul><li>Provides a strong and stable base for the vertebral column</li><li>Permits the trunk of the body to twist and bend in almost all directions</li></ul>

Sources: OpenStax (2018); Standring (2016); Vleeming et al. (2012)

Range of motion

The hip joint allows a wide range of motion. The motion is enabled by the pelvic muscles that wield three degrees of freedom on three reciprocally perpendicular axes. The most common types of motion include flexion, extension, internal and external rotation, abduction, adduction and hyperextension (Cheatham, Hanney and Kolber 2017; Moreno-Pérez *et al.* 2016). The greatest motion occurs at the external pelvic platform. Table 9.2 summarises the estimated ranges of motion in the hip for weight-training participants.

Table 9.2. Hip range of motion values for recreational weight-training participants

	Right hip	Left hip	p-value
Flexion	120.4±14.5°	121.3±13.8°	0.50
Extension	12.6±5.9°	12.6±7.6°	0.95
Internal rotation	36.4±9.5°	36.1±8.7°	0.82
External rotation	32.2±8.7°	32.0±9.4°	0.78
Abduction	42.6±11.3°	43.2±12.3°	0.64

Source: Cheatham et al. *(2017)*

The SIJ has a limited range of motion in contrast to the hip. Although in past times many in the medical community believed it to be immobile, studies have demonstrated rotation of less than 4° and translation of up to 1.6 mm (Laslett 2008).

Common injuries

A major injury to the pelvis and the sacrum is often caused by a fall, motor vehicle accident, violent activity, sporting accident or penetrating trauma. These injuries are common in all populations, including male and female, the very young and old, and athletes of numerous sports (Larkin 2010) (see Table 9.3).

Table 9.3. Common injuries of the pelvis and sacrum

Common injuries	Incidence	Characteristics
Pelvic fracture	• 37 cases per 100,000 person-years (USA) • 19 cases per 100,000 person-years (UK)	• Typically, a fracture of the bony structures of the pelvic region that often includes the hip bone, sacrum and coccyx • Often results from traumatic events such as road traffic accidents or falls • The severity of pelvic fractures varies along a continuum from mild to life-threatening as a function of the amount of force applied
Sacroiliac joint dysfunction	• Accounts for 13–30% of back pain cases	• Commonly refers to anomalous position or movement of SIJ structures that may or may not result in pain • Can result from motor vehicle accidents, falls or other traumatic events that apply force to the SIJ region • Common indications include pain in the lower back, buttock(s), hip or groin as well as a sensation of numbness, sciatic leg pain and a frequent urge to urinate
Hip dislocation	• Accounts for 5% of traumatic joint dislocations	• Usually results from dissipation of a large amount of energy directed along the axis of the femur • Posterior dislocations are the most common (>90%) but may also be anterior or central • Motor vehicle accidents are implicated in a majority of cases • May be associated with fractures of the femoral head or neck

Sources: Foulk and Mullis (2010); Johansen et al. (1997); Laslett (2008); Rashbaum et al. (2016); Russell and Jarett (2018); Schmidt, Sciulli and Altman (2005)

Red flags

It is always important for therapists to check for red flag symptoms as these may indicate emergent medical conditions requiring immediate attention (Kahn and Xu 2017) (see Table 9.4). While individual red flags do not necessarily point to a specific pathology, they have great utility in outlining the need for further investigation. Multiple red flags, when present, do require further investigation (Airaksinen *et al.* 2006).

Table 9.4. Red flags for serious pathology in the pelvis and sacrum

Condition	Signs and symptoms
Pathologic femoral neck fractures	• Elderly females (>70 years) with hip, groin or upper thigh pain • Severe, constant hip, groin or knee pain that worsens with motion • History of trauma such as a blunt force to the upper thigh or falling from a standing position
Osteonecrosis of the femoral head	• History of prolonged use of corticosteroids • History of trauma • History of alcohol abuse • History of slipped capital femoral epiphysis • Slow, consistent onset of pain • Pain in the groin, thigh or knee that increases with load bearing
Cancer	• Past or present history of malignancy (e.g., prostate, breast or any reproductive cancer) • Family history of cancers of the pelvic region (e.g., colon, prostate or any reproductive cancer) • Rectal disturbances and bowel anomalies (e.g., bleeding in the rectal/anal region, black stool) • Chronic, localised, progressive pain independent of position
Infection	• Fever, chills • History of infections of the urinary tract or skin • Burning sensation when urinating • Persistent pain at rest • No recovery following six weeks of conventional therapy
Slipped capital femoral epiphysis	• Obese adolescent • History of trauma • Pain in the groin that increases with weight bearing • Limited internal rotation and abduction of the hip resulting in the involved leg being held in external rotation
Legg–Calvé–Perthes disease	• Young boy (aged 5–8) with groin/thigh pain • Antalgic gait • Pain intensified with abduction, internal rotation or other movements of the hip

Sources: Boissonnault (2005); Gabbe et al. (2009); Gibbons and Tehan (2006); Henschke, Maher and Refshauge (2007); Meyers et al. (2000); Reiman et al. (2014); van den Bruel et al. (2010)

Special tests

Table 9.5 is not an exhaustive list of special tests but gives you, the therapist, a guide for this area. If you are unsure of the interpretation of any test that you complete with your patient, we advise that you refer to the most appropriate medical professional for further investigations.

Table 9.5. Special tests for pelvis and SIJ dysfunction

Test	Procedure	Positive sign	Interpretation	Test statistics
Trendelenburg test	The patient stands facing the therapist. The therapist then asks the patient to transfer their weight to the affected leg while slowly raising the unaffected foot off the ground, flexing both the hip and knee. The therapist observes the movement as the weight is shifted towards the symptomatic side	• Pelvis drops on the non-weight-bearing side (i.e., hemipelvis falls below the horizontal)	✓ Gluteal dysfunction ✓ Hip subluxation or dislocation	Specificity: 0.76 Sensitivity: 0.72
Patrick or FABER test	The patient assumes a supine posture with one leg extended and the test leg is placed in a flexed, abducted, externally rotated (FABER) position. The therapist gently applies overpressure of the hip by pressing the test leg knee towards the table while stabilising the anterior superior iliac spine (ASIS)	• Pain elicited on the groin/ ipsilateral side anteriorly	✓ Hip joint dysfunction	Specificity: 0.71 Sensitivity: 0.57
		• Pain elicited on the buttock/ contra-lateral side posteriorly	✓ SIJ irritation	
Gaenslen's test	The patient assumes either a supine or side-lying posture. The therapist asks the patient to draw both legs up onto their chest before slowly lowering the test leg into extension	• SIJ pain	✓ SIJ dysfunction	Specificity: 0.26 Sensitivity: 0.71
Ober test	The patient assumes a side-lying position with the test leg on top. The affected knee is flexed to 90° and the therapist passively abducts and pulls the patient's upper leg posteriorly, until the thigh is in line with the torso	• Leg remains in abduction and fails to fall to the table	✓ Extreme tension of the iliotibial band	Specificity: 0.98 Sensitivity: 0.13

Test	Procedure	Positive sign	Interpretation	Test statistics
Thomas test	The patient begins the procedure seated at the edge of the foot of the treatment table. The therapist then guides the patient into a supine posture with the knees and hips fully flexed With the non-test leg in full flexion, the therapist guides the test leg into hip extension. The therapist then flexes the test leg to 90°	• Straight leg lifting off the treatment table	✓ Flexion contracture of the hip	Specificity: 0.92 Sensitivity: 0.89
Log roll test	The patient lies supine with both lower limbs extended. The therapist passively rotates both fully extended legs medially and laterally to end range	• A painful sensation in the anterior hip or groin	✓ Intraarticular hip pathology ✓ Piriformis syndrome ✓ Slipped capital femoral epiphysis	Specificity: 0.33 Sensitivity: 1.00
Femoral nerve tension test (Ely's test)	The patient lies prone while the therapist passively flexes the test leg to 90° before lifting the hip into full extension. The therapist monitors the ipsilateral hip for uplift from the table	• Ipsilateral hip flexion and anterior rotation of the pelvis	✓ Irritation of femoral nerve ✓ Rectus femoris contracture	Specificity: 1.00 Sensitivity: 0.63

Sources: Douglas, Nicol and Robertson (2013); Ganderton et al. (2017); Goodman and Snyder (2013); Gross, Fetto and Rosen (2016); Hattam and Smeatham (2010); Kahn and Xu (2017); Lee et al. (2015); Magee (2014); Olson (2016); Rahman et al. (2013); Reiman et al. (2013)

References

Airaksinen, O., Brox, J.I., Cedraschi, C., Hildebrandt, J., Klaber-Moffett, J., Kovacs, F. *et al.* (2006) 'European guidelines for the management of chronic nonspecific low back pain.' *European Spine Journal 15*, s192–s300. Available at https://doi.org/10.1007/s00586-006-1072-1

Boissonnault, W.G. (2005) *Primary Care for the Physical Therapist.* St Louis, MO: Elsevier Saunders. Available at https://doi.org/10.1016/B978-0-7216-9659-1.X5001-1

Cheatham, S., Hanney, W.J. and Kolber, M.J. (2017) 'Hip range of motion in recreational weight training participants: A descriptive report.' *International Journal of Sports Physical Therapy 12*, 764–773. Available at https://doi.org/10.16603/ijspt20170764

Cohen, S.P., Chen, Y. and Neufeld, N.J. (2013) 'Sacroiliac joint pain: A comprehensive review of epidemiology, diagnosis and treatment.' *Expert Review of Neurotherapeutics 13*, 99–116. Available at https://doi.org/10.1586/ern.12.148

Douglas, G., Nicol, F. and Robertson, C. (eds) (2013) *Macleod's Clinical Examination*. 13th edn. London: Churchill Livingstone Elsevier.

Ernst, E. (2007) 'Adverse effects of spinal manipulation: A systematic review.' *Journal of the Royal Society of Medicine 100*, 330–338. Available at https://doi.org/10.1258/jrsm.100.7.330

Foulk, D.M. and Mullis, B.H. (2010) 'Hip dislocation: Evaluation and management.' *Journal of the American Academy of Orthopaedic Surgeons 18*, 199–209. Available at https://doi.org/10.5435/00124635-201004000-00003

Gabbe, B.J., Bailey, M., Cook, J.L., Makdissi, M. *et al.* (2009) 'The association between hip and groin injuries in the elite junior football years and injuries sustained during elite senior competition.' *British Journal of Sports Medicine 44*(1), 799–802.

Ganderton, C., Semciw, A., Cook, J. and Pizzari, T. (2017) 'Demystifying the clinical diagnosis of greater trochanteric pain syndrome in women.' *Journal of Women's Health 26*, 633–643. Available at https://doi.org/10.1089/jwh.2016.5889

Gibbons, P. and Tehan, P. (2006) *Manipulation of the Spine, Thorax and Pelvis: An Osteopathic Perspective*. 2nd edn. Philadelphia, PA: Churchill Livingstone/Elsevier.

Goldflies, M., Rosen, M. and Hauser, B. (2018) 'Benefits of mechanical manipulation of the sacroiliac joint: A transient synovitis case study.' *Journal of Orthopaedic Research 2*. Available at https://doi.org/10.31031/OPROJ.2018.02.000542

Goodman, C.C. and Snyder, T.E.K. (2013) *Differential Diagnosis for Physical Therapists: Screening for Referral*. 5th edn. St Louis, MO: Elsevier Saunders.

Gross, J.M., Fetto, J. and Rosen, E. (2016) *Musculoskeletal Examination*. 4th edn. Chichester: John Wiley & Sons Ltd.

Hattam, P. and Smeatham, A. (2010) *Special Tests in Musculoskeletal Examination: An Evidence-based Guide for Clinicians*. Philadelphia, PA: Churchill Livingstone Elsevier.

Henschke, N., Maher, C.G. and Refshauge, K.M. (2007) 'Screening for malignancy in low back pain patients: A systematic review.' European Spine Journal 16(10), 1673–1679.

Johansen, A., Evans, R.J., Stone, M.D., Richmond, P.W., Lo, S.V. and Woodhouse, K.W. (1997) 'Fracture incidence in England and Wales: A study based on the population of Cardiff.' *Injury 28*, 655–660. Available at https://doi.org/10.1016/S0020-1383(97)00144 7

Kahn, S.B. and Xu, R.Y. (2017) *Musculoskeletal Sports and Spine Disorders: A Comprehensive Guide*. Cham, Switzerland: Springer. Available at https://doi.org/10.1007/978-3-319-50512-1

Kamali, F. and Shokri, E. (2012) 'The effect of two manipulative therapy techniques and their outcome in patients with sacroiliac joint syndrome.' *Journal of Bodywork and Movement Therapies 16*, 29–35. Available at https://doi.org/10.1016/j.jbmt.2011.02.002

Larkin, B. (2010) 'Epidemiology of Hip and Pelvis Injury.' In P.H. Seidenberg and J.D. Bowen (eds) *The Hip and Pelvis in Sports Medicine and Primary Care*. New York: Springer.

Laslett, M. (2008) 'Evidence-based diagnosis and treatment of the painful sacroiliac joint.' *The Journal of Manual & Manipulative Therapy 16*, 142–152. Available at https://doi.org/10.1179/jmt.2008.16.3.142

Lee, S.Y., Sung, K.H., Chung, C.Y., Lee, K.M., Kwon, S.S., Kim, T.G. *et al.* (2015) 'Reliability and validity of the Duncan-Ely test for assessing rectus femoris spasticity in patients with cerebral palsy.' *Developmental Medicine & Child Neurology 57*, 963–968. Available at https://doi.org/10.1111/dmcn.12761

Magee, D.J. (2014) *Orthopedic Physical Assessment*. 6th edn. St Louis, MO: Saunders.

Meyers, W.C., Foley, D.P., Garrett, W.E., Lohnes, J.H. and Mandlebaum, B.R. (2000) 'Management of severe lower abdominal or inguinal pain in high-performance athletes.' *American Journal of Sports Medicine 28*(1), 2–8.

Moreno-Pérez, V., Ayala, F., Fernandez-Fernandez, J. and Vera-Garcia, F.J. (2016) 'Descriptive profile of hip range of motion in elite tennis players.' *Physical Therapy in Sport 19*, 43–48. Available at https://doi.org/10.1016/j.ptsp.2015.10.005

Olson, K.A. (2016) *Manual Physical Therapy of the Spine*. 2nd edn. St Louis, MO: Elsevier.

OpenStax (2018) *Anatomy and Physiology*. OpenStax College. Available at https://openstax.org/details/books/anatomy-and-physiology

Rahman, L.A., Adie, S., Naylor, J.M., Mittal, R., So, S. and Harris, I.A. (2013) 'A systematic review of the diagnostic performance of orthopedic physical examination tests of the hip.' *BMC Musculoskeletal Disorders 14*, 257. Available at https://doi.org/10.1186/1471-2474-14-257

Rashbaum, R.F., Ohnmeiss, D.D., Lindley, E.M., Kitchel, S.H. and Patel, V.V. (2016) 'Sacroiliac joint pain and its treatment.' *Journal of Spinal Disorders & Techniques 29*, 42–48. Available at https://doi.org/10.1097/BSD.0000000000000359

Reiman, M.P., Goode, A.P., Hegedus, E.J., Cook, C.E. and Wright, A.A. (2013) 'Diagnostic accuracy of clinical tests of the hip: A systematic review with meta-analysis.' *British Journal of Sports Medicine 47*, 893–902. Available at https://doi.org/10.1136/bjsports-2012-091035

Russell, G.V. and Jarett, C.A. (2018) 'Pelvic fractures: Background.' Medscape. Available at https://emedicine.medscape.com/article/1247913-overview

Schmidt, G.L., Sciulli, R. and Altman, G.T. (2005) 'Knee injury in patients experiencing a high-energy traumatic ipsilateral hip dislocation.' *The Journal of Bone and Joint Surgery – Series A 87*, 1200–1204. Available at https://doi.org/10.2106/JBJS.D.02306

Standring, S. (ed.) (2016) *Gray's Anatomy: The Anatomical Basis of Clinical Practice.* 41st edn. New York: Elsevier.

van den Bruel, A., Haj-Hassan, T., Thompson, M., Buntinx, F., Mant, D. and European Research Network on Recognising Serious Infection investigators (2010) 'Diagnostic value of clinical features at presentation to identify serious infection in children in developed countries: A systematic review.' *The Lancet 375* (9717), 834–845.

Vleeming, A., Schuenke, M.D., Masi, A.T., Carreiro, J.E., Danneels, L. and Willard, F.H. (2012) 'The sacroiliac joint: An overview of its anatomy, function and potential clinical implications.' *Journal of Anatomy 221* (6), 537–567. Available at https://doi.org/10.1111/j.1469-7580.2012.01564.x

WHO (World Health Organization) (2005) *WHO Guidelines on Basic Training and Safety in Chiropractic.* Geneva: WHO.

HIP MANIPULATION TECHNIQUES

Supine proximal femoral head manipulation

- Ask the patient to lie supine with their head supported using a pillow.

- Flex the patient's hip to 90° and fully flex the knee.

- Place a towel over their upper thigh, as shown.

- Interlace your fingers around the thigh with the ulnar border over the joint line.

- Ask the patient to inhale and exhale.

- As the patient exhales, increase hip flexion while distracting the hip to engage the barrier.

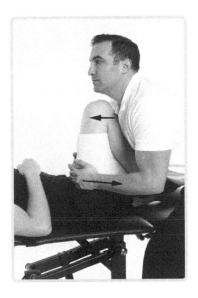

- On the engagement of the barrier, perform the manipulation by pulling your hands towards you.

Key to note:

- If the patient cannot flex the knee, rest the knee on you shoulder bent ideally to 90° or whatever the patient can manage.

- You may want to place a towel over the midline of the body for modesty and the addition of a barrier.

- If you are unable to interlace your fingers around the patient's upper thigh as shown, use a towel and hold both ends.

- You can add bias to internal and external rotation by placing the hip into either position and perform the technique the same way, as described above.

- Remember not to keep the patient at the barrier for too long.

Supine proximal femur manipulation with external rotation

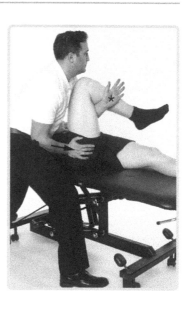

- Ask the patient to lie supine with their head supported using a pillow.

- Flex the affected hip to approximately 90° or as much as they possibly can.

- Stand with an asymmetrical stance, as shown.

- Your left hand enters the medial aspect of the distal femur and exits at the proximal lateral tibia.

- Your right hand contacts the proximal femoral head, as shown.

- Externally rotate the affected hip until you engage the barrier.

- Ask the patient to inhale and exhale.

- As the patient exhales, engage the barrier by creating external rotation of the affect hip.

- On the engagement of the barrier, perform the manipulation by pushing the proximal head of the femur oblique and inferior, as shown.

Key to note:

- You may want to place a towel over the patient's adductors as a barrier and a broader contact for you to push against.

- You can perform this technique for bias towards internal rotation by switching the directions shown.

- Remember not to keep the patient at the barrier for too long.

Prone proximal femoral head manipulation

- Ask the patient to lie prone.

- Flex the knee to 90° and place your hand underneath the knee, as shown.

- With your other hand contact the posterior aspect of the femoral head via your thenar eminence.

- Ask the patient to inhale and exhale.

- As the patient exhales, engage the barrier by creating extension of the femur, lifting the hip into extension via the knee while pushing down onto the femoral head.

- On the engagement of the barrier, perform the manipulation by pushing down on the femoral head.

Key to note:

- You may want to place a towel over the patient's proximal femur and knee.

- You can add bias to internal and external rotation by placing the hip into either position and perform the technique the same way as described above.

- Remember not to keep the patient at the barrier for too long.

Prone proximal femoral head manipulation

- Ask the patient to lie in the prone position.

- Externally rotate the affected hip and rest the patient's knee on your thigh, as shown.

- Contact the posterior-lateral aspect of the femoral head via your thenar eminence while the other hand supports the knee resting on your thigh, as shown.

- Ask the patient to inhale and exhale.

- As the patient exhales, engage the barrier by pressure in an oblique direction on the proximal femoral head while the other hand lifts the patient's knee superior, creating abduction.

- On the engagement of the barrier, perform the manipulation by pushing down on the femoral head in an inferior and oblique direction, as shown.

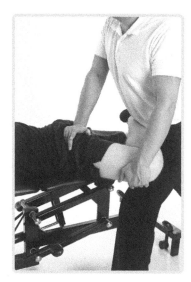

Key to note:

- Externally rotate the affected hip within a comfortable position for the patient.

- You may want to place a towel over the patient's proximal femur and your thigh to create a barrier and increase comfort for the patient.

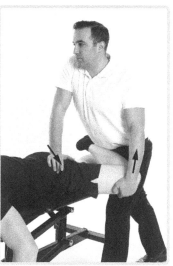

- Remember not to keep the patient at the barrier for too long.

Side-lying proximal femoral head manipulation

- The patient will be in the side-lying position with a towel between their knees flexed at 90°.

- Contact the greater trochanter of the affected side via your thenar eminence.

- Ask the patient to inhale and exhale.

- As the patient exhales, engage the barrier by creating inferior pressure down the line of the femur.

Key to note:

- Remember not to keep the patient at the barrier for too long.

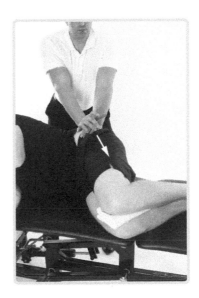

Side-lying proximal femoral head manipulation with external rotation

- The patient will be in the side-lying position with a towel between their knees flexed at 90°.

- Use one hand to contact the proximal-lateral aspect of the femur via your thenar eminence while the other contacts the medial aspect of the knee, as shown.

- Create abduction and external rotation via the hand in contact with the medial aspect of the knee, as shown.

- Simultaneously, your other hand contacting the proximal femur applies pressure in an inferior and oblique direction, as shown.

- Ask the patient to inhale and exhale.

- As the patient exhales, engage the barrier by creating inferior pressure down the line of the femur and abduction and external rotation of the hip.

- Once the barrier is engaged, complete the manipulation through the hand contacting the proximal femur in an inferior and oblique direction, as shown.

Key to note:

- Do not rush this technique.

- Be sure to position the table at the correct height.

- Remember not to keep the patient at the barrier for too long.

Supine proximal femur manipulation with compression and internal rotation

- The patient lies supine with their head supported using a pillow.

- Flex the affected hip to approximately 90° or as much as they possibly can.

- Stand with an asymmetrical stance, as shown.

- Your right hand contacts the knee as shown; with your bodyweight, add compression downwards.

- Your left hand contacts the calcaneum, as shown.

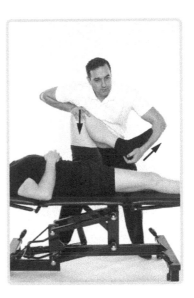

- Compress and internally rotate the affected hip until you engage the barrier.

- Ask the patient to inhale and exhale.

- As the patient exhales, engage the barrier by creating compression and internal rotation of the affected hip.

- On the engagement of the barrier, perform the manipulation by rotating the hip via your left hand, holding the calcaneus in a rotating direction.

Key to note:

- You may want to add a towel onto the knee to avoid direct compression to the patella.

- Your left hand controls the foot into a neutral position to maintain the hip position.

- You can perform this technique for bias towards external rotation by switching the directions shown.

- Remember not to keep the patient at the barrier for too long.

Unilateral pubis manipulation with hip extension

- The patient lies supine with their head supported using a pillow.

- Stand with an asymmetrical stance, as shown.

- The patient needs to hold the affected hip into flexion for support.

- Place the affected side limb off the table with the hip moving into extension.

- Place one hand just lateral to the pubis of the affected side (use a towel for a barrier and comfort, as shown).

- Your right hand contacts the knee, as shown, and prevents the hip from moving into internal and external rotation.

- Ask the patient to inhale and exhale.

- As the patient exhales, engage the barrier dropping your bodyweight through the hand in contact with the knee while restricting the pubis.

- On the engagement of the barrier, perform the manipulation by dropping your bodyweight through your right hand, as shown.

Key to note:

- Make sure the patient lies as close to you as possible.

- If the patient cannot reach their knee, place a towel around their hamstring and get them to hold the hip in flexion via the towel.

- Avoid too much pressure over the pubis.

- Remember not to keep the patient at the barrier for too long.

10

KNEE, ANKLE AND FOOT

Introduction

Manipulative therapy may be used as an adjunct to conventional treatment approaches for the lower limbs. The modern reality, with an increased scope of work-related musculoskeletal injuries, has played a role in the development of new multimodal, manipulative treatment approaches for lower extremity dysfunction (Hoskins *et al.* 2006). Manipulative therapy, being non-invasive, has proved to be quite desirable for patients with certain knee pathologies. Studies on the effects of manipulative techniques on the knee have demonstrated that manipulation is effective in pain reduction for osteoarthritic patients while causing little to no discomfort for the individuals (James *et al.* 2018; Pollard 2000). Additional benefits of manipulation for knee conditions, as highlighted in recent literature, include greater mobility and reduced stiffness, among others (James *et al.* 2018; Salamh *et al.* 2017).

Ankle injuries are among the most frequent clinical problems affecting a large cross-section of the population, and non-invasive treatments would be appealing to many patients (López-Rodríguez *et al.* 2007). Several studies have reported the potential benefits of joint manipulation for people diagnosed with various pathological conditions of the ankle. In a review exploring the efficacy of manipulative therapy on ankle injuries, Loudon, Reiman and Sylvain (2014) reported that 'manual therapy techniques are beneficial in restoring or improving dorsiflexion, posterior talar glide, stride speed and step length and force distribution of the foot' (pp.365–70). Brandolini *et al.* (2019) demonstrated, using a specific manipulative technique, that ankle manipulation was also effective in improving range of motion, alleviating symptoms and preventing recurrent injury in athletes. Such benefits are potentially life-changing for athletes who suffer career-threatening ankle injuries in active sports.

Along with knee and ankle treatment, manipulative therapy has shown many positive benefits, with few drawbacks, for individuals with foot problems. While the commonly expected musculoskeletal benefits of manipulation would apply to the foot region, some studies have demonstrated further advantages in the context of regional interdependence. Foot manipulation has been shown to have potential application in the treatment of pregnancy-related pelvic girdle pain (Melkersson *et al.* 2017). These examples, while briefly touching on a few applications of manipulative therapy for the lower extremity and beyond, serve to highlight how far we have come, and show the bright prospects for the future.

This chapter will be a useful resource for therapists in the diagnosis of pathological conditions of the lower extremity with a special focus on the knee, ankle and foot. The chapter includes an overview of the joints in these regions of the lower limb, their ranges of motion, common injuries and red flags for manipulative therapy. Special tests for knee, ankle and foot dysfunction are also outlined.

Joints

The knee joint is a bicompartmental synovial joint in human anatomy and is the largest in the human body (see Table 10.1). The joint occurs between the femur and the tibia bones. The joint also includes articulation between the patella and femur. The tibia and fibula articulate with each other at the superior and inferior tibiofibular joints. All bones of the knee except the fibula play a role in movement (Standring 2016).

Inferior to the knee joint is the talocrural joint (ankle joint). This joint is formed by the distal ends of the tibia and fibula 'gripping' the talus. Within the foot there are multiple joints that may be classified topographically based on whether they are in the hindfoot, midfoot or forefoot. These joints perform various complex movements required as the foot fulfils its functional roles as a platform for standing and for shock absorption and propulsion in gait (Magee *et al.* 2016).

Table 10.1. Joints of the knee, ankle and foot

Joint name	Description	Function
Knee joint	• A bicompartmental synovial (modified hinge) joint • Forms a complex hinge between three bones, the femur, tibia and patella • Consists of different joints: tibiofemoral, between the tibia and femur; patellofemoral, between the femur and the patella; superior tibiofibular, between the tibia and fibula • Enclosed by a single articular capsule that enfolds the entire joint complex	• Allows flexion and extension of the leg • Ensures weight-bearing support of the body • Allows transmission of bodyweight in vertical and horizontal directions • Superior tibiofibular joint allows slight gliding motion • Tolerates minor degree of internal and external rotation when flexed

Joint name	Description	Function
Tibiofemoral joint	• A synovial (modified hinge) joint • Connects between the medial and lateral condyles of the femur and the tibial condyles of the tibia • Reinforced by two wedge-shaped articular discs, the medial and lateral meniscus	• Assists as the weight-bearing joint of the knee • Permits flexion and extension of the leg • Allows some medial and lateral rotation of the leg
Patellofemoral joint	• A diarthrodial plane joint • Articulates the anterior and distal part of the femur with the patella (kneecap) • Consists of the posterior surface of the patella and the trochlear surface of the distal anterior femur	• Provides stability and strength to the knee joint • Conveys tensile forces generated by the quadriceps to the patellar tendon • Increases the lever arm of the extensor mechanism • Permits the knee to straighten when standing • Helps to perform the activities of daily living (walking, cycling, stair climbing, jogging and squatting)
Proximal tibiofibular joint	• A diarthrodial plane joint between the medial facet of the head of the fibula and the tibial facet on the posterolateral tibial condyle • Has a fibrous capsule strengthened by anterior and posterior superior tibiofibular ligaments and tendinous insertions, making it intrinsically stable when the knee is stretched	• Allows twisting movements of the leg • Disperses torsional stresses applied at the ankle • Transfers load between the feet and the body • Dissipates lateral tibial bending movements
Distal tibiofibular joint	• A syndesmotic joint • Formed by joining the distal end of the fibula with the lateral side of the tibia • Is supported by the strong interosseus ligament	• The inferior segment assists in stabilising the tibiofibular syndesmosis • Permits slight movements for the lateral malleolus to rotate laterally when the ankle dorsiflexes • Helps to uphold the ankle joint integrity

Ankle or talocrural joint	• A hinge joint between the distal ends of the tibia and fibula and the trochlea of the talus • Is reinforced by strong ligamentous structures that provide stability to the ankle • Surrounded by loose connective tissue called paratenon • Is maintained by the shape of the talus and its tight fit between the tibia and fibula, in a neutral position	• Facilitates rotation about an axis of rotation • Permits dorsiflexion and plantar flexion movements via axis in talus
Subtalar or talocalcaneal joint	• A joint formed by two bones in the foot, the talus and calcaneus (heel bone) • Includes three articulations between the talus and calcaneus: anterior, middle and posterior	• Allows internal and external rotation of the foot
Talocalcaneonavicular joint	• A joint between the navicular, talus and calcaneus bones • Comprises two articulations, a frontal talocalcaneal and a talonavicular	• Allows pronation and supination of the foot
Calcaneocuboid joint	• A joint formed between the calcaneus and the cuboid bone • Strengthened by bifurcate, long plantar and plantar calcaneocuboid ligaments	• Allows minor gliding movements between the calcaneus and the cuboid bone
Tarsometatarsal or Lisfranc joints	• Arthrodial joints • Formed between the bones of the second row of the tarsus and the bases of the metatarsal bones • Stabilised by strong interosseus dorsal and plantar ligaments	• Allow small gliding movements at the feet
Intermetatarsal joints	• Robust synovial joints • Involve articulations between the bases of the 2nd to 5th metatarsal bones • Interosseus dorsal and plantar ligaments provide strength	• Allow slight gliding movements at the feet

Joint name	Description	Function
Metatarsophalangeal joints	• Ovoid joints formed between the heads of the metatarsal bones and the bases of the proximal phalanges • Reinforced by collateral, deep transverse metatarsal and plantar ligaments	• Permit a variety of movements at the toes, including flexion, extension, abduction, adduction and circumduction
Interphalangeal joints	• Ginglymoid (hinge) joints • Articulations between the phalanges of the toes • Subdivided into two sets of articulations: proximal interphalangeal joints and distal interphalangeal joints	• Allow limited flexion and extension of the medial and distal phalanges

Sources: Giangarra and Manske (2017); Magee et al. (2016); Norkin and White (2009); Standring (2016)

Range of motion

Knee

The knee joint consists of three major ligaments, namely, the patella, collateral and cruciate ligaments. These ligaments provide strength and stability for the knee to perform such functions as weight-bearing support of the body and transmission of bodyweight in perpendicular and plane directions (Standring 2016). The movements allowed by the joint include extension, flexion, minor lateral and medial rotation and a slight gliding motion as allowed by the superior tibiofibular joint (see Tables 10.2 and 10.3). These movements make it possible for the knee to perform daily normal activities such as walking, cycling, stair climbing, standing, sitting, jogging and squatting. The range of motion of the knee is typically measured by using either a hand or radiographic goniometry (Peters *et al.* 2011).

Table 10.2. Normal range of motion of the knee

Movement type	Range of motion
Flexion	138–158°
Extension	5–10°
Lateral rotation (knee flexed 90°)	30–40°
Medial rotation (knee flexed 90°)	10°

Sources: Peters et al. (2011); Soucie et al. (2011)

Table 10.3. Normative ranges of motion of the knee in different age groups

Age	Motion	Mean range of motion	
		Males	Females
2–8 years	Flexion	147.8°	152.6°
	Extension	1.6°	5.4°
9–19 years	Flexion	142.2°	142.3°
	Extension	1.8°	2.4°
20–44 years	Flexion	137.7°	141.9°
	Extension	1.0°	1.6°
45–69 years	Flexion	132.9°	137.8°
	Extension	0.5°	1.2°

Source: Soucie et al. (2011)

Ankle

The ankle is a hinge joint between the distal ends of the tibia and fibula and the trochlea of the talus. The joint enables rotation about an axis of rotation and permits dorsiflexion and plantar flexion movements via the axis in the talus (Young *et al.* 2013). See Table 10.4 for approximate ranges of motion for the ankle joint.

Table 10.4. Approximate range of motion of the ankle

Movement type	Range of motion
Normal dorsiflexion	0–50°
Normal plantar flexion	0–20°
Dorsiflexion, knee extended	14–48°
Dorsiflexion, knee flexed	16–60°

Source: Brockett and Chapman (2016)

Foot

The foot is divided into three divisions, namely, the rearfoot, midfoot and forefoot. It functions to support bodyweight, provide balance, absorb shock and transfer ground reaction forces. Various joints are found on the foot including talocrural, subtalar, midtarsal, tarsometatarsal, metatarsophalangeal and interphalangeal joints. The joints display different types of motion (see Table 10.5). The talocrural joint allows for dorsiflexion and plantar flexion movements in the sagittal plane while the subtalar joint permits pronation and supination movements. The midtarsal joint allows inversion and eversion and flexion and extension. The metatarsophalangeal joint provides motion in the sagittal and transverse plane with flexion, extension, adduction and abduction motions. The interphalangeal joints allow motion in the sagittal plane, allowing pure flexion and extension (Brockett and Chapman 2016).

Table 10.5. Range of motion of the foot joints

Joint name	Movement type	Range of motion
Subtalar joint	Inversion	0–50°
	Eversion	0–26°
Metatarsophalangeal joints	Flexion (great toe)	0–45°
	Extension (great toe)	0–80°
	Flexion (lesser toes)	0–40°
	Extension (lesser toes)	0–70°
Interphalangeal joints	Flexion (great toe)	0–90°
	Flexion (lesser toes)	0–30°
	Extension (great toe and other toes)	0–80°

Sources: Blackwood et al. *(2005); Norkin and White (2009); Oatis (1988)*

Common injuries

Injuries to the knee, ankle and foot are among the most frequent musculoskeletal injuries occurring in all demographic groups. These injuries are often attributed to trauma resulting from sporting accidents, falling from a height, road traffic accidents or violent activity, to name but a few. Due to frequent overuse of the lower extremity in sporting activities, athletes often injure their ankles, feet or knees, and this may result in short- or long-term disability leading to potential loss of productivity and income. The most common injuries of the knee, ankle and foot are summarised in Table 10.6 below.

Table 10.6. Common injuries of the knee, ankle and foot

Common injuries	Incidence	Characteristics
Anterior cruciate ligament sprain	• 68.6 per 100,000 person-years (USA) • 8.06 per 100,000 person-years (UK)	• A very frequent knee injury • The anterior cruciate ligament is torn, usually with a 'pop', resulting in knee instability • Higher incidence in athletes participating in sports such as American football, soccer, tennis, downhill skiing, volleyball and basketball that put a lot of strain on the knees • Associated with sudden directional changes of the lower extremity, or sudden stops from running • May also occur with high load landing from a jump • Half of these injuries may result in damage to other knee structures (e.g., meniscus, articular cartilage, other ligaments)
Medial collateral ligament sprain	• 24 per 100,000 person-years (USA) • 5.21 per 100,000 person-years (UK)	• Another high-frequency knee injury • The medial collateral ligament that prevents the knee from bending inward is torn • Frequently associated with athletes in contact sports (e.g., American football, rugby, wrestling, judo, rugby, hockey) • Often occurs due to a hit or direct blow to the outer aspect of the knee • Usually occurs after rapid directional changes while running as well as bending or twisting the lower extremity • May include a 'popping' noise accompanied by pain, swelling and tenderness around the knee
Meniscal tear	• 61 per 100,000 person-years (USA) • 23.76 per 100,000 person-years (UK)	• Meniscal tears are very common injuries of the knee • The rubbery fibrocartilaginous meniscus, with a cushioning role in the knee, is ruptured • The highest incidence is in athletes participating in contact sports • Normally results from strong, rapid twisting or hyperflexion of the knee joint • Characterised by strong pain, inflammation and tenderness in the knee area • May occur with a 'popping' sound

Common injuries	Incidence	Characteristics
Patellar tendinopathy (Jumper's knee)	• 0.88 per 10,000 athlete exposures (USA) • 0.12 injuries per 1000 hours among elite athletes (UK)	• This is a painful injury associated with overuse of the patellar tendon • Pain is activity-related and is often located below the patella, in the proximal region of the tendon • Occurs most frequently in jumping athletes • Short-term overuse may result in a reactive tendon that normalises with load adjustment, but high load may lead to chronic injury
Ankle sprain	• 215 per 100,000 person-years (USA) • 52.7–60.9 per 10,000 people (UK)	• Reported as the most common ankle injury • The ankle ligaments are stretched beyond their limits and in some cases they may rupture • Athletes who frequently participate in running and jumping sports are at highest risk for ankle sprains • The injury may be short-term with complete recovery, or it may result in long-term disability
Plantar fasciitis	• 10.5 per 1000 person-years (USA)	• This degenerative disease of the plantar fascia results in stabbing pain at the heel and plantar side of the foot • It is estimated to affect a tenth of the population at some point in their lifetime, with the most commonly affected demographic being middle-aged people • Inconsistent leg length, nerve entrapment, muscle tightness, excessive pronation, over-training and uncomfortable footwear are recognised risk factors for plantar fasciitis
Peroneal tendonitis	• 35% of asymptomatic cases	• An injury resulting from ankle overuse with pain at the lateral portion • The peroneal tendons are inflamed • Frequently affects athletes involved in sports with repetitive ankle motion, excessive eversion and pronation

Sources: Bliss (2017); Bollen (2000); Bridgman (2003); Clayton and Court-Brown (2008); Davda et al. (2017); De Vries et al. (2017); Gans et al. (2018); Khan et al. (2018); Pedowitz, O'Connor and Akeson (2003); Raj and Bubnis (2018); Reinking (2016); Sanders et al. (2016); Santana and Sherman (2018); Scher et al. (2009); Swenson et al. (2013); Waterman et al. (2010)

Red flags

It is good practice for therapists to familiarise themselves with the red flags for serious pathology in the lower extremity before pursuing manipulative interventions (WHO 2005). Red flag symptoms help therapists identify potentially serious pathology early, and exercise sound clinical judgement to avert any potential harm to the patient. Whenever a combination of the red flags in Table 10.7 is observed, manual therapists should refer patients for further clinical screening.

Table 10.7. Red flags for serious pathology in the knee, ankle and foot

Condition	Signs and symptoms
Knee fracture	• History of recent trauma to the knee • Intense localised swelling with effusion and ecchymosis • Severe tenderness along the joint line • Flexion less than 90° • Patient unable to walk more than four weight-bearing steps
Compartment syndrome	• History of blunt trauma • Cumulative trauma • Overuse • Intense, persistent pain and firmness to anterior shin compartment • Reduced pulse • Paraesthesia • Pain with toe dorsiflexion • Intense pain associated with stretch on affected muscles
Extensor mechanism disruption	• Quadriceps or patella tendon rupture • Superior translation of the patella
Fractures	• Trauma from a motor vehicle accident, blunt force to the ankle or a fall • Inflammation on affected leg with concomitant pain • Relentless synovitis • Involved tissues feel sore and are highly sensitive • Difficulty walking more than four weight-bearing steps
Deep vein thrombosis (DVT)	• Recent surgery, period of limited mobility, pregnancy or malignancy • Hot, erythemic and very tender calf • Fever and malaise • Positive Homans sign • Pain exaggerated with use of the extremity (e.g., walking or standing) and diminished with rest

Condition	Signs and symptoms
Septic arthritis	• Fever and chills accompanied by consistent pain • History of bacterial infection • Recent invasive medical intervention (e.g., surgery or injection) • Open wound • Joint inflammation with no history of trauma • General malaise or loss of appetite • Compromised immunity
Cancer	• Chronic pain with no history of trauma • History of malignancy • Weight loss with no clear explanation • General malaise with or without fever and weakness • Presence of swelling or unexplained presence of tumours and deformity

Sources: Boissonnault (2005); Magee (2014); Stephenson (2013); Wise (2015)

Special tests

Table 10.8 is not an exhaustive list of special tests but gives you, the therapist, a guide for this area. If you are unsure of the interpretation of any test that you complete with your patient, we advise that you refer to the most appropriate medical professional for further investigations.

Table 10.8. Special tests for knee, ankle and foot dysfunction

Test	Procedure	Positive sign	Interpretation	Test statistics
Lachman/ Trillat/ Ritchie test	In this one-plane test, the patient assumes a supine posture. The patient's foot is stabilised between the therapist's thigh and the table. With the therapist's outside hand stabilising the femur, they apply gentle force, pulling the tibia forward, with the intent of generating anterior translation	• Excessive anterior excursion of the tibia on the femur accompanied by a soft or absent joint end-feel • Diminishing of the normal slope of the infrapatellar tendon	✓ Anterior cruciate ligament injury ✓ May also indicate injury to the posterior oblique ligament or arcuate-popliteus complex	Specificity: 0.91 Sensitivity: 0.86

Posterior drawer test	With the patient lying supine, the hip and knee are flexed at 45° and 90° respectively with the tibia in neutral rotation. The therapist pushes backwards on the tibia after stabilising the patient's foot	• Posterior movement of the tibia relative to the femur	✓ Posterior cruciate ligament laxity	Specificity: 0.99 Sensitivity: 0.90
Abduction/ valgus stress test	In this one-plane medial instability assessment the therapist pushes the patient's knee medially (valgus stress) while stabilising the ankle in slight lateral rotation. The knee is typically in full extension and 30° flexion The test thigh may be rested on the table to help the patient relax	• Medial collateral ligament laxity on application of valgus stress	✓ Injury to posterior and medial cruciate ligaments	Specificity: not reported Sensitivity: 0.91
McMurray's test	The patient assumes a supine position with the knee in full flexion. The therapist rotates the tibia medially while extending the knee The therapist repeatedly changes the amount of flexion while applying medial rotation then extension to the tibia to test the complete posterior aspect of the meniscus (i.e., posterior horn to middle segment)	• A snap or click accompanied by pain	✓ Loose meniscal fragment	Specificity: 0.93 Sensitivity: 0.59
Talar tilt test	The patient lies supine or on their side with the foot relaxed. The normal side is tested first to establish a point of comparison. With the therapist holding the foot at 90°, the talus is tilted from side to side into inversion and eversion	• An increased talar tilt or joint laxity when compared with the normal side	✓ Torn calcaneofibular ligament	Specificity: 0.74 Sensitivity: 0.52

Test	Procedure	Positive sign	Interpretation	Test statistics
Thompson's/ Simmonds' test	The patient assumes a prone position or kneels on a chair with the feet hanging over the edge. With the patient relaxed, the therapist squeezes the calf muscles	• Absence of plantar flexion when the calf muscle is squeezed	✓ Achilles tendon rupture	Specificity: 0.93 Sensitivity: 0.96
Anterior drawer test	With the patient lying prone, the ankle in a neutral position and the foot in 20° of plantar flexion, the therapist applies an anteriorly directed force to the calcaneus. This may also be done by pushing backwards on the tibia	• Increased anterior translation compared with the normal side	✓ Anterior talocrural joint laxity	Specificity: 0.38 Sensitivity: 0.74
Kleiger test (external rotation stress test)	The patient is seated, while flexing the knee at 90°. The therapist stabilises the leg with one hand and applies a passive lateral rotational stress externally to the affected foot and ankle	• Significant pain at the anterolateral part of the distal tibiofibular syndesmosis	✓ Syndesmotic injury ✓ Deltoid ligament injury	Specificity: 0.85 Sensitivity: 0.20

Sources: Boissonnault (2005); Croy et al. (2013); de César, Ávila and de Abreu (2011); Douglas, Nicol and Robertson (2013); Hattam and Smeatham (2010); Magee (2014); Malanga et al. (2003); Manske and Prohaska (2008); Ostrowski (2006); Schwieterman et al. (2013); Slaughter et al. (2014); Wise (2015)

References

Blackwood, C.B., Yuen, T.J., Sangeorzan, B.J. and Ledoux, W.R. (2005) 'The midtarsal joint locking mechanism.' *Foot & Ankle International 26*, 1074–1080. Available at https://doi.org/10.1177/107110070502601213

Bliss, J.P. (2017) 'Anterior cruciate ligament injury, reconstruction, and the optimization of outcome.' *The Indian Journal of Orthopaedics 51*, 606–613. Available at https://doi.org/10.4103/ortho.IJOrtho_237_17

Boissonnault, W.G. (2005) *Primary Care for the Physical Therapist*. St Louis, MO: Elsevier Saunders. Available at https://doi.org/10.1016/B978-0-7216-9659-1.X5001-1

Bollen, S. (2000) 'Epidemiology of knee injuries: Diagnosis and triage.' *British Journal of Sports Medicine 34*, 227–228.

Brandolini, S., Lugaresi, G., Santagata, A., Ermolao, A., Zaccaria, M., Marchand, A.M. *et al.* (2019) 'Sport injury prevention in individuals with chronic ankle instability: Fascial Manipulation® versus control group: A randomized controlled trial.' *Journal of Bodywork and Movement Therapies* 23(2), 316–323. Available at https://doi.org/10.1016/J.JBMT.2019.01.001

Bridgman, S.A. (2003) 'Population-based epidemiology of ankle sprains attending accident and emergency units in the West Midlands of England, and a survey of UK practice for severe ankle sprains.' *Emergency Medicine Journal* 20, 508–510. Available at https://doi.org/10.1136/emj.20.6.508

Brockett, C.L. and Chapman, G.J. (2016) 'Biomechanics of the ankle.' *Journal of Orthopaedic Trauma* 30, 232–238. Available at https://doi.org/10.1016/j.mporth.2016.04.015

Clayton, R.A.E. and Court-Brown, C.M. (2008) 'The epidemiology of musculoskeletal tendinous and ligamentous injuries.' *Injury* 39, 1338–1344. Available at https://doi.org/10.1016/j.injury.2008.06.021

Croy, T., Koppenhaver, S., Saliba, S. and Hertel, J. (2013) 'Anterior talocrural joint laxity: Diagnostic accuracy of the anterior drawer test of the ankle.' *Journal of Orthopaedic & Sports Physical Therapy* 43, 911–919. Available at https://doi.org/10.2519/jospt.2013.4679

Davda, K., Malhotra, K., O'Donnell, P., Singh, D. and Cullen, N. (2017) 'Peroneal tendon disorders.' *EFORT Open Reviews* 2, 281–292. Available at https://doi.org/10.1302/2058-5241.2.160047

de César, P.C., Ávila, E.M. and de Abreu, M.R. (2011) 'Comparison of magnetic resonance imaging to physical examination for syndesmotic injury after lateral ankle sprain.' *Foot & Ankle International* 32, 1110–1114. Available at https://doi.org/10.3113/FAI.2011.1110

De Vries, A.J., Koolhaas, W., Zwerver, J., Diercks, R.L., Nieuwenhuis, K., van der Worp, H. *et al.* (2017) 'The impact of patellar tendinopathy on sports and work performance in active athletes.' *Research in Sports Medicine* 25, 253–265. Available at https://doi.org/10.1080/15438627.2017.1314292

Douglas, G., Nicol, F. and Robertson, C. (eds) (2013) *Macleod's Clinical Examination.* 13th edn. London: Churchill Livingstone Elsevier.

Gans, I., Retzky, J.S., Jones, L.C. and Tanaka, M.J. (2018) 'Epidemiology of recurrent anterior cruciate ligament injuries in national collegiate athletic association sports: The Injury Surveillance Program, 2004–2014.' *Orthopaedic Journal of Sports Medicine* 6, 2325967118777782. Available at https://doi.org/10.1177/2325967118777823

Giangarra, C.E. and Manske, R.C. (2017) *Clinical Orthopaedic Rehabilitation: A Team Approach.* Philadelphia, PA: Elsevier.

Hattam, P. and Smeatham, A. (2010) *Special Tests in Musculoskeletal Examination: An Evidence-based Guide for Clinicians.* London: Churchill Livingstone Elsevier.

Hoskins, W., McHardy, A., Pollard, H., Windsham, R. and Onley, R. (2006) 'Chiropractic treatment of lower extremity conditions: A literature review.' *Journal of Manipulative and Physiological Therapies* 29, 658–671. Available at https://doi.org/10.1016/j.jmpt.2006.08.004

James, D.A., Nigrini, C.M., Manske, R.C. and Caughran, A.T. (2018) 'The Arthritic Knee.' In C.E. Giangarra, R.C. Manske and S.B. Brotzman (eds) *Clinical Orthopaedic Rehabilitation: A Team Approach.* Philadelphia, PA: Elsevier.

Khan, T., Alvand, A., Prieto-Alhambra, D., Culliford, D.J., Judge, A., Jackson, W.F. *et al.* (2018) 'ACL and meniscal injuries increase the risk of primary total knee replacement for osteoarthritis: A matched case-control study using the Clinical Practice Research Datalink (CPRD).' *British Journal of Sports Medicine* 53, 15, 1–5. Available at https://doi.org/10.1136/bjsports-2017-097762

López-Rodríguez, S., de-las-Peñas, C.F., Alburquerque-Sendín, F., Rodríguez-Blanco, C. and Palomeque-del-Cerro, L. (2007) 'Immediate effects of manipulation of the talocrural joint on stabilometry and baropodometry in patients with ankle sprain.' *Journal of Manipulative and Physiological Therapies* 30, 186–192. Available at https://doi.org/10.1016/j.jmpt.2007.01.011

Loudon, J.K., Reiman, M.P. and Sylvain, J. (2014) 'The efficacy of manual joint mobilisation/manipulation in treatment of lateral ankle sprains: A systematic review.' *British Journal of Sports Medicine* 48, 365–370. Available at https://doi.org/10.1136/bjsports-2013-092763

Magee, D.J. (2014) *Orthopedic Physical Assessment*. 6th edn. St Louis, MO: Saunders.

Magee, D.J., Zachazewski, J.E., Quillen, W.S. and Manske, R.C. (2016) *Pathology and Intervention in Musculoskeletal Rehabilitation*. 2nd edn. Maryland Heights, MO: Elsevier. Available at https://doi.org/10.1016/c2012-0-05970-4

Malanga, G.A., Andrus, S., Nadler, S.F. and McLean, J. (2003) 'Physical examination of the knee: A review of the original test description and scientific validity of common orthopedic tests.' *Archives of Physical Medicine and Rehabilitation* 84, 592–603. Available at https://doi.org/10.1053/apmr.2003.50026

Manske, R.C. and Prohaska, D. (2008) 'Physical examination and imaging of the acute multiple ligament knee injury.' *North American Journal of Sports Physical Therapy* 3, 191–197.

Melkersson, C., Nasic, S., Starzmann, K. and Bengtsson Boström, K. (2017) 'Effect of foot manipulation on pregnancy-related pelvic girdle pain: A feasibility study.' *Journal of Chiropractic Medicine* 16, 211–219. Available at https://doi.org/10.1016/j.jcm.2017.05.003

Norkin, C.C. and White, D.J. (2009) *Measurement of Joint Motion: A Guide to Goniometry*. Philadelphia, PA: F.A. Davis.

Oatis, C.A. (1988) 'Biomechanics of the foot and ankle under static conditions.' *Physical Therapy* 68, 1815–1821.

Ostrowski, J.A. (2006) 'Accuracy of 3 diagnostic tests for anterior cruciate ligament tears.' *Journal of Athletic Training* 41, 120–121.

Pedowitz, R.A., O'Connor, J.J. and Akeson, W.H. (eds) (2003) *Daniel's Knee Injuries: Ligament and Cartilage Structure, Function, Injury, and Repair*. 2nd edn. Philadelphia, PA: Lippincott Williams & Wilkins.

Peters, P.G., Herbenick, M.A., Anloague, P.A., Markert, R.J. and Rubino, L.J. (2011) 'Knee range of motion: Reliability and agreement of 3 measurement methods.' *American Journal of Orthopaedics* 40, E249–E252.

Pollard, H.P. (2000) 'The Effect of Chiropractic Manual Therapy on the Spine, Hip and Knee.' University of Wollongong Thesis Collection.

Raj, M.A. and Bubnis, M.A. (2018) 'Knee Meniscal Tears.' StatPearls. Available at http://knowledge.statpearls.com/chapter/np-adult/23936

Reinking, M.F. (2016) 'Current concepts in the treatment of patellar tendinopathy.' *The International Journal of Sports Physical Therapy* 11(6), 854–866.

Salamh, P., Cook, C., Reiman, M.P. and Sheets, C. (2017) 'Treatment effectiveness and fidelity of manual therapy to the knee: A systematic review and meta-analysis.' *Musculoskeletal Care* 15, 238–248. Available at https://doi.org/10.1002/msc.1166

Sanders, T.L., Maradit Kremers, H., Bryan, A.J., Larson, D.R., Dahm, D.L., Levy, B.A. *et al.* (2016) 'Incidence of anterior cruciate ligament tears and reconstruction.' *American Journal of Sports Medicine* 44, 1502–1507. Available at https://doi.org/10.1177/0363546516629944

Santana, J.A. and Sherman, A.I. (2018) 'Jumpers Knee.' StatPearls. Available at www.ncbi.nlm.nih.gov/books/NBK532969

Scher, C.D.L., Belmont, L.C.P.J., Bear, M.R., Mountcastle, S.B., Orr, J.D. and Owens, M.B.D. (2009) 'The incidence of plantar fasciitis in the United States military.' *The Journal of Bone & Joint Surgery (American volume)* 91, 2867–2872. Available at https://doi.org/10.2106/JBJS.I.00257

Schwieterman, B., Haas, D., Columber, K., Knupp, D. and Cook, C. (2013) 'Diagnostic accuracy of physical examination tests of the ankle/foot complex: A systematic review.' *International Journal of Sports Physical Therapy* 8, 416–426.

Slaughter, A.J., Reynolds, K.A., Jambhekar, K., David, R.M., Hasan, S.A. and Pandey, T. (2014) 'Clinical orthopedic examination findings in the lower extremity: Correlation with imaging studies and diagnostic efficacy.' *RadioGraphics* 34, e41–e55. Available at https://doi.org/10.1148/rg.342125066

Soucie, J.M., Wang, C., Forsyth, A., Funk, S., Denny, M., Roach, K.E. *et al.* (2011) 'Range of motion measurements: Reference values and a database for comparison studies.' *Haemophilia* 17, 500–507. Available at https://doi.org/10.1111/j.1365-2516.2010.02399.x

Standring, S. (ed.) (2016) *Gray's Anatomy: The Anatomical Basis of Clinical Practice*. 41st edn. New York: Elsevier.

Stephenson, C. (2013) *The Complementary Therapist's Guide to Red Flags and Referrals*. London: Churchill Livingstone.

Swenson, D.M., Collins, C.L., Best, T.M., Flanigan, D.C., Fields, S.K. and Comstock, R. (2013) 'Epidemiology of knee injuries among US high school athletes, 2005/2006–2010/2011.' *Medicine & Science in Sports & Exercise* 45, 462–469. Available at https://doi.org/10.1249/MSS.0b013e318277acca

Waterman, B., Owens, B., Davey, S., Zacchilli, M. and Belmont, P. (2010) 'The epidemiology of ankle sprains in the United States.' *Journal of Bone & Joint Surgery* (*American volume*) 92, 2279–2284. Available at https://doi.org/10.2106/JBJS.I.01537

WHO (World Health Organization) (2005) *WHO Guidelines on Basic Training and Safety in Chiropractic*. Geneva: WHO.

Wise, C.H. (2015) *Orthopaedic Manual Physical Therapy: From Art to Evidence*. Philadelphia, PA: F.A. Davis Company.

Young, R., Nix, S., Wholohan, A., Bradhurst, R. and Reed, L. (2013) 'Interventions for increasing ankle joint dorsiflexion: A systematic review and meta-analysis.' *Journal of Foot and Ankle Research* 6, 46. Available at https://doi.org/10.1186/1757-1146-6-46

KNEE MANIPULATION TECHNIQUES

Supine fibula head thrust, bilateral hand contact

- The patient is in a supine position.

- Stand on the side of the affected limb, facing the patient.

- Bend the patient's knee and hip to 90°.

- With your right hand, move the lower leg towards the patient's gluteal in a superior-inferior (SI) direction until you reach full knee flexion and the back of the contact hand is in contact with the tissues of the distal hamstrings.

- Place your left hand around the lateral aspect of the knee so that the 1st MCP joint is in contact with the posterior aspect of the proximal fibula head and the fingers are resting gently in the popliteal fossa; your right hand is contacting the posterior aspect of the knee, moving away the soft tissue.

- With both hands, move the lower leg towards the patient's gluteal in an SI direction until you reach full knee flexion and the back of the contact hand is in contact with the tissues of the distal hamstrings.

- The right arm will contact the tibia and allow you to lean against it, adding slight internal rotation.

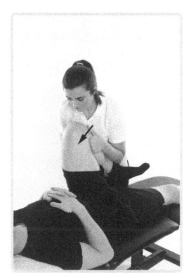

Set-up for the knee and knee thrust

- Ask the patient to inhale and exhale.

- At the end of the exhalation, engage the barrier by leaning forwards and manipulate the fibula head anteriorly-posteriorly (AP).

Prone fibula head thrust, pisiform hand contact

- The patient is in a prone position.

- Stand on the side of the affected limb, facing the patient.

- Bend the patient's knee and hip to 90°.

- Pisiform contact of the lateral aspect of the fibula head, with the other hand rotating the foot outwards.

- Build the pre-tension, and when the barrier is reached, a short thrust towards the hamstring is applied.

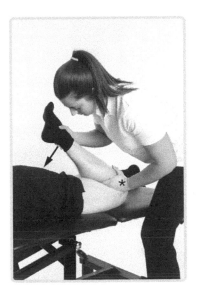

Prone fibula head thrust, MCP contact

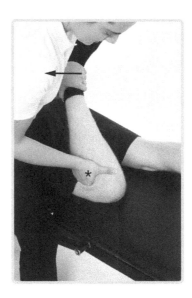

- The patient is in a prone position.

- Stand on the side of the affected limb, facing away from the patient.

- Bend the patient's knee and hip to 90°.

- With the lateral hand, use an MCP contact of the lateral aspect of the fibula head, with the other hand rotating the foot outwards.

- Build the pre-tension, and when the barrier is reached, a short thrust towards the hamstring is applied.

Prone fibula head thrust, forearm contact

- The patient is in a prone position.

- Stand on the side of the affected limb, facing away from the patient.

- Bend the patient's knee and hip to 90°.

- With the lateral arm, place the forearm in contact of the lateral aspect of the fibula head, with the other hand rotating the foot outwards.

- Build the pre-tension, and when the barrier is reached, a short thrust towards the hamstring is applied.

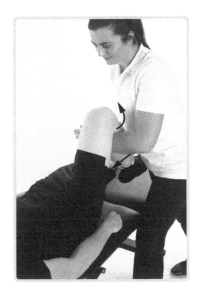

Prone knee thrust, posterior to anterior glide of the left tibiofemoral joint

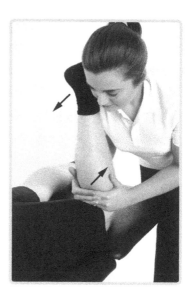

- The patient is in a prone position.

- Stand on the side of the affected limb, facing away from the patient.

- Bend the patient's knee and hip to 90°.

- Stand by the affected knee at the side of the table, and bend forwards so you can rest the patient's foot on your inside shoulder.

- Use both hands to contact the posterior aspect of the proximal tibia.

- Create a knife-edge contact with both hands, and now lean forwards and traction your hands back to create pre-tension.

- With both hands, once you have removed the articular slack, use a long lever axis to thrust the proximal tibia backwards, gapping the joint.

Supine knee thrust, traction thrust for the tibiofemoral joint

- The patient is in a supine position.

- Stand on the side of the affected limb, facing the patient.

- Bring the patient's leg off the table and place it between your thighs, to create a lock using compression.

- Use both hands to contact the inferior aspect of the knee on the proximal tibia.

- Locking both hands, now lean backwards and traction your hands back to create pretension.

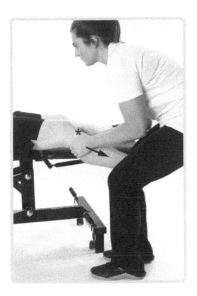

- With both hands, once you have removed the articular slack, use a long lever axis to thrust the proximal tibia backwards, gapping the joint.

Medial to lateral and lateral to medial thrust of the right tibiofemoral joint

- The patient is in a supine position.

- Stand on the side of the affected limb, facing the patient.

- Bring the patient's leg off the table and place it between your thighs to create a lock using compression.

- This technique will be for either the medial or lateral tibiofemoral joint, so change hands accordingly to the affected side.

- Your supporting hand contacts the inferior aspect of the knee on the proximal tibia.

- Your thrusting hand contacts either the medial or lateral of the distal femur. Now lean backwards and traction your hands back to create pre-tension.

- Once you have removed the tissue slack, creating pre-manipulation tension, use a short thrust for the tibiofemoral joint, either medially or laterally.

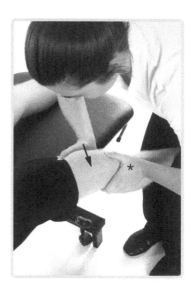

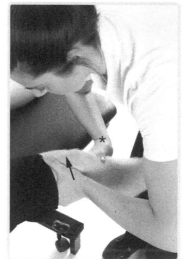

Prone knee thrust, traction thrust for the tibiofemoral joint

- The patient is in a prone position.

- Stand at the end of the table and take hold of the affected limb.

- Ensure the knee remains in contact with the table and, with both hands, hold the lower leg above the medial and lateral malleoli and raise the leg up by 30°.

- Create a lock using both hands.

- Locking both hands, lean backwards and traction your hands back to create pre-tension.

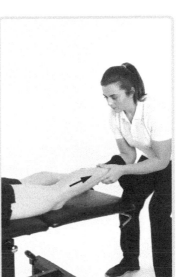

- Once you have removed the tissue slack, creating pre-manipulation tension, use a long lever axis to complete a traction thrust to move the proximal tibia backwards.

Supine proximal tibia anterior thrust

- The patient is in a supine position.

- Stand at the side of the table and take hold of the affected limb.

- Bring the knee up to 90°, ensuring the foot remains in contact with the table; stabilise this by sitting on the foot if needed.

- Create a lock using both hands behind the tibia, underneath the knee joint.

- Locking both hands, lean backwards and traction your hands back to create pre-tension.

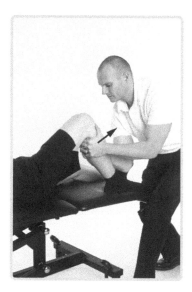

- Once you have removed the tissue slack, creating pre-manipulation tension, use a short lever axis to complete a thrust anteriorise the proximal tibia forwards.

Supine proximal tibia thrust posterior, wedge technique

- The patient is in a supine position.

- Stand at the side of the table and take hold of the affected limb.

- Place a wedge underneath the knee to reduce movement, and allow the thrust to be directed towards the tibia.

- Create a lock using both hands in front of the tibia, underneath the knee joint.

- Locking both hands, lean forwards to create pre-tension.

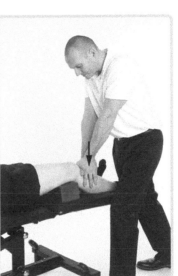

- Once you have removed the tissue slack, creating pre-manipulation tension, use a long lever axis to complete a traction thrust to move the proximal tibia backwards.

FOOT AND ANKLE MANIPULATION TECHNIQUES

Supine cuneiform manipulation

- The patient is lying in the supine position.

- Maintain an asymmetrical stance, as shown.

- Clasp your hands together on the anterior and posterior aspect of the target cuneiform, as shown.

- Ask the patient to inhale and then slowly exhale.

- As the patient starts to exhale, begin to build the barrier inferiorly.

- At the engagement of the barrier, provide manipulation in the direction shown.

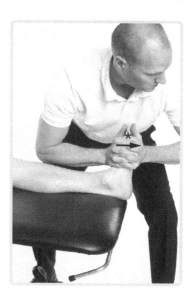

Key to note:

- The patient's foot is kept as close to neutral as possible.

- Try to keep your elbows as close to you as possible.

- Wait for the patient to complete the breathing cycle.

- Do not use excessive force – you will not need it.

Supine tibio-talar manipulation

- The patient is lying in the supine position.

- Adopt an asymmetrical stance, as shown.

- Using both hands, contact just below the medial and lateral malleolus.

- The pads of your thumbs should make contact with the trochlea of the talus.

- Ask the patient to inhale and then slowly exhale.

- As the patient starts to exhale, stabilise the target by clasping your hands together, as shown, and create traction.

- At the end of exhalation, apply the manipulation in the direction shown.

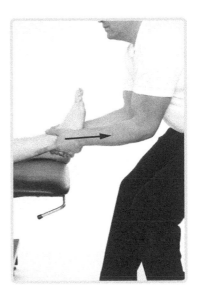

Key to note:

- You ideally need to keep the patient's foot in a neutral position.

- This technique can be completed in prone and lying on the side.

- Remember to use your legs in order to limit the force from your arms.

- Try to keep your elbows as close to you as possible.

Metatarsal head manipulation

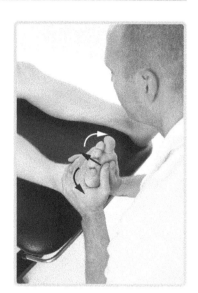

- The patient is lying in the supine position.

- Adopt an asymmetrical stance.

- Interlace your fingers over the metatarsal head.

- Your thumbs can add plantar or dorsi flexion as needed.

- Ask the patient to inhale and then slowly exhale.

- As the patient starts to exhale, begin to engage the barrier in the direction as shown.

- At the end of exhalation, the barrier should be engaged; apply the manipulation in the direction shown.

Key to note:

- Remember to use your legs in order to limit the force from your arms.

- Try to keep your elbows as close to you as possible.

- Do not use excessive force – you will not need it.

Supine talus manipulation

- The patient is lying in the supine position, with their knee in flexion.

- Adopt an asymmetrical stance, as shown.

- Your hand stabilises the medial and lateral malleolus.

- Your other hand contacts the trochlea of the talus in the direction shown.

- Ask the patient to inhale and then slowly exhale.

- As the patient starts to exhale, add your pressure in an oblique direction to engage the barrier.

- At the end of exhalation, the barrier should be engaged; perform your manipulation in the direction shown.

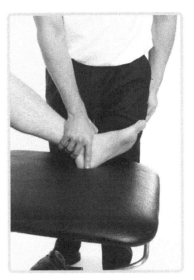

Key to note:

- You can support the lateral aspect of the foot with your leg, as shown.

- Try to keep your elbows as close to you as possible.

- Wait for the patient to complete the breathing cycle.

- Do not use excessive force – you will not need it.

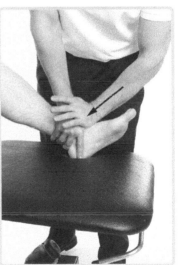

Supine navicular manipulation

- The patient is lying in the supine position with their knee in flexion and calcaneus in contact with the table.

- Adopt an asymmetrical stance, as shown.

- Your left thumb makes contact on the superior aspect of the navicular, reinforced by the pisiform from your right hand.

- Ask the patient to inhale and then slowly exhale.

- As the patient starts to exhale, add pressure in an oblique direction to engage the barrier.

- At the end of exhalation, the barrier should be engaged; perform your manipulation in the direction shown.

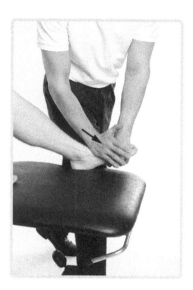

Key to note:

- You can support the lateral aspect of the foot with your leg, as shown.

- Try to keep your elbows as close to you as possible.

- Wait for the patient to complete the breathing cycle.

- Do not use excessive force – you will not need it.

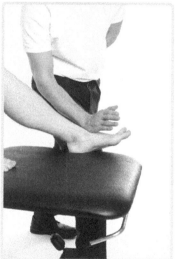

Medial cuneiform and 1st metatarsal manipulation

- The patient is lying in the prone position with their knee in flexion, with the lateral of the foot held, as shown, against your abdomen.

- Adopt an asymmetrical stance, as shown.

- Your thenar eminence stabilises the medial aspect of the foot, while your thumb applies static pressure to the cuneiform.

- Your other hand grasps the 1st metatarsal, as shown.

- Ask the patient to inhale and then slowly exhale.

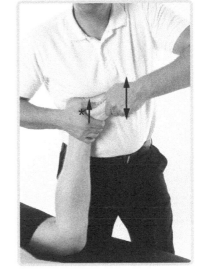

- As the patient starts to exhale, begin to build the barrier.

- At the end of exhalation, the barrier should be engaged; perform your manipulation in the direction shown.

Key to note:

- Place a small towel between the patient's foot and your abdomen to give a stable contact on the plantar aspect.

- Try to keep your elbows as close to you as possible.

- Wait for the patient to complete the breathing cycle.

- Do not use excessive force – you will not need it.

Supine navicular manipulation with extended leg

- The patient is lying in the supine position with their knee in full extension for stability.

- Adopt an asymmetrical stance, as shown.

- Locate and hold the navicular, as shown.

- With your contact hand, locate and hold the navicular, as shown.

- Ask the patient to inhale and then slowly exhale.

- As the patient starts to exhale, begin to build the barrier.

- At the end of exhalation, the barrier should be engaged; perform your manipulation in the direction shown.

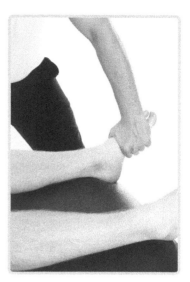

Key to note:

- You can place a bolster under the knee if needed.

- The foot is kept in neutral.

- Try to keep your elbows as close to you as possible.

- Wait for the patient to complete the breathing cycle.

- Do not use excessive force – you will not need it.

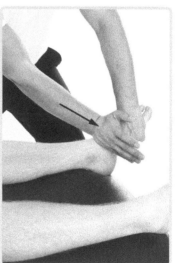

Side-lying navicular manipulation with knee in flexion

- The patient is lying in the supine position with their knee in flexion and the hip externally rotated.

- Adopt an asymmetrical stance.

- Locate and hold the first metatarsal, as shown.

- Your other hand via the pisiform contacts the navicular tubercle, as shown.

- Ask the patient to inhale and then slowly exhale.

- As the patient starts to exhale, begin to build the barrier by rotating the 1st metatarsal towards you and pushing the navicular oblique towards the table.

- At the end of exhalation, the barrier should be engaged; perform your manipulation in the direction shown via the contact hand on the navicular.

Key to note:

- Do not leave the patient in external rotation of the hip for too long.

- You can place a towel under the foot for more comfort.

- The foot is kept in neutral.

- Try to keep your elbows as close to you as possible.

- Wait for the patient to complete the breathing cycle.

- Do not use excessive force – you will not need it.

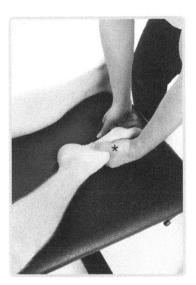

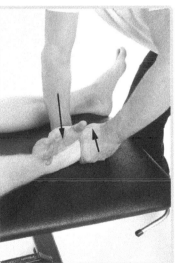

Proximal 1st metatarsal with knee flexion

- The patient is lying in the supine position with their knee in flexion.

- Adopt an asymmetrical stance.

- Locate the proximal head of the 1st metatarsal and make contact via the pisiform, as shown.

- Using the web of your free hand, make contact on your hand, as shown.

- Ask the patient to inhale and then slowly exhale.

- As the patient starts to exhale, begin to build the barrier by adding downward pressure through your top hand.

- At the end of exhalation, the barrier should be engaged; perform your manipulation in the direction shown.

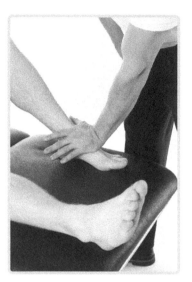

Key to note:

- You can place a towel under the foot for more comfort.

- The foot is kept as close to neutral as possible.

- Avoid this position if the patient has an Achilles tendon problem.

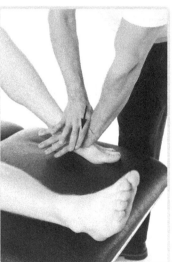

- Try to keep your elbows as close to you as possible.

- Wait for the patient to complete the breathing cycle.

- Do not use excessive force – you will not need it.

Hallux manipulation

- The patient is lying in the supine position with their knee in extension.

- Take hold of the hallux with one hand, as shown.

- With your other hand, contact the joint line of the 1st metatarsal.

- Ask the patient to inhale and then slowly exhale.

- As the patient starts to exhale, begin to build the barrier in the direction shown.

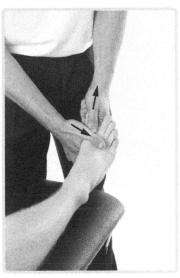

- At the end of exhalation, the barrier should be engaged; perform your manipulation in the transverse direction along the line of the 1st metatarsal, as shown.

Key to note:

- The foot is kept as close to neutral as possible.

- Try to keep your elbows as close to you as possible.

- Wait for the patient to complete the breathing cycle.

- Do not use excessive force – you will not need it.

Calcaneum manipulation in prone

- The patient is lying in the prone position.

- Maintain an asymmetrical stance position.

- Stabilise the lower leg with one hand while the other contacts with the posterior aspect of the calcaneus, as shown.

- Ask the patient to inhale and then slowly exhale.

- As the patient starts to exhale, begin to build the barrier by applying pressure in the direction shown.

- At the end of exhalation, the barrier should be engaged; perform your manipulation in the direction shown.

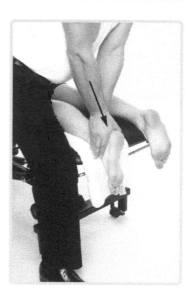

Key to note:

- Using a towel as shown makes this technique much more comfortable.

- Use your legs to transfer the force.

- The foot is kept as close to neutral as possible.

- Try to keep your elbows as close to you as possible.

- Wait for the patient to complete the breathing cycle.

- Do not use excessive force – you will not need it.

Tibio-talar manipulation

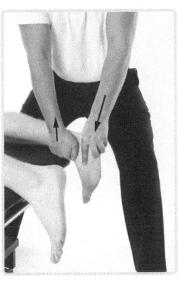

- The patient is lying in the prone position.

- Maintain an asymmetrical stance position.

- Stabilise the lower leg with one hand while the other contacts with the posterior aspect of the calcaneus, as shown.

- Ask the patient to inhale and then slowly exhale.

- As the patient starts to exhale, begin to build the barrier by applying pressure in the directions shown.

- At the end of exhalation, the barrier should be engaged; perform your manipulation by pulling the tibia towards you while simultaneously pushing the calcaneus down.

Key to note:

- Keep your arms straight and use your legs to transfer the force.

- The foot is kept as close to neutral as possible.

- Try to keep your elbows as close to you as possible.

- Wait for the patient to complete the breathing cycle.

- Do not use excessive force – you will not need it.

Talocrural manipulation

- The patient is lying in the prone position.

- Maintain an asymmetrical stance position.

- Make contact on the trochlea of the talus and calcaneus, as shown.

- Ask the patient to inhale and then slowly exhale.

- As the patient starts to exhale, begin to build the barrier by applying traction towards you.

- At the end of exhalation, the barrier should be engaged; perform your manipulation by pulling the talus and calcaneus towards you.

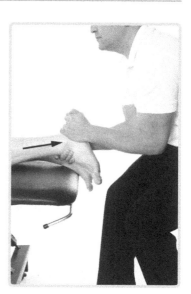

Key to note:

- This technique can be completed in supine and side-lying.

- The foot is kept as close to neutral as possible.

- Try to keep your elbows as close to you as possible.

- Wait for the patient to complete the breathing cycle.

- Do not use excessive force – you will not need it.

Cuneiform manipulation

- The patient is lying in the supine position.

- Maintain an asymmetrical stance position.

- Make contact on the posterior aspect of the calcaneus while making contact on the target cuneiform, as shown.

- Ask the patient to inhale and then slowly exhale.

- As the patient starts to exhale, begin to build the barrier by stabilising the calcaneus and pushing the cuneiform in the direction shown.

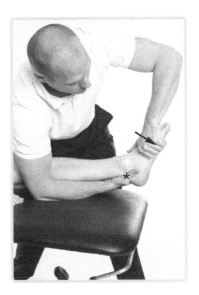

Key to note:

- The foot is kept as close to neutral as possible.

- Try to keep your elbows as close to you as possible.

- Wait for the patient to complete the breathing cycle.

- Do not use excessive force – you will not need it.

Cuboid manipulation

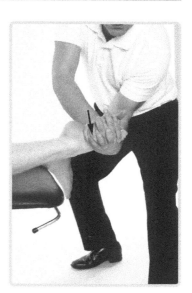

- The patient is lying in the prone position.

- Maintain an asymmetrical stance position.

- Make contact on the posterior aspect of the cuboid with your thumb, which is reinforced by the pisiform, as shown.

- Ask the patient to inhale and then slowly exhale.

- As the patient starts to exhale, begin to build the barrier by plantar flexing the foot while adding downward pressure.

- Once the barrier is engaged, perform the manipulation in the direction shown via the pisiform contact.

Key to note:

- Try to keep your elbows as close to you as possible.

- Wait for the patient to complete the breathing cycle.

- Do not use excessive force – you will not need it.

Cuboid manipulation pisiform contact

- The patient is lying in the prone position.

- Maintain an asymmetrical stance position.

- Your left hand controls the dorsal aspect of the foot while the ulnar border of your right hand makes contact on the posterior aspect of the cuboid.

- Ask the patient to inhale and then slowly exhale.

- As the patient starts to exhale, begin to build the barrier by plantar flexing the foot while adding downward pressure.

- Once the barrier is engaged, perform the manipulation in the direction shown via the pisiform contact.

Key to note:

- Try to keep your elbows as close to you as possible.

- Wait for the patient to complete the breathing cycle.

- Do not use excessive force – you will not need it.

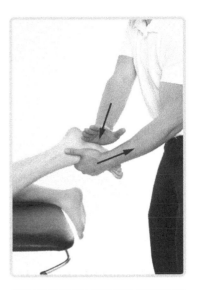

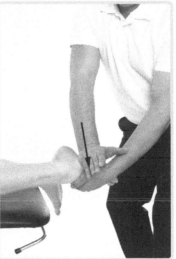

Cuboid manipulation thumb content

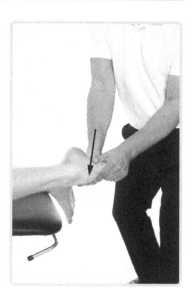

- The patient is lying in the prone position.

- Maintain an asymmetrical stance position.

- Using both hands, contact the dorsal aspect of the target foot and cross your thumbs over the posterior aspect of the target cuboid, as shown.

- Ask the patient to inhale and then slowly exhale.

- As the patient starts to exhale, begin to build the barrier by plantar flexing the foot while adding downward pressure through your thumbs.

- Once the barrier is engaged, perform the manipulation in the direction shown.

Key to note:

- Crossing the thumbs over gives the sensation of a broader contact than you are using.

- Try to keep your elbows as close to you as possible.

- Wait for the patient to complete the breathing cycle.

- Do not use excessive force – you will not need it.

Glossary

Abduction Movement of an outlying joint away from the midline.

AC joint Acromioclavicular joint.

Adduction Movement of an outlying joint towards the midline.

Amplitude Distance of articulation.

Anterior Near or toward the front.

Anteroposterior (AP) Direction from front to back.

AP Anteroposterior.

Applicator Part of the therapist's body that is placed on the contact point of the patient.

Articular or periarticular adhesions Grade 1 is identified as a filmy or silk-like adhesion connecting the inter-synovial structures from the roof to the bottom structure.

Grade 2 is commonly observed in the anterolateral aspect of the upper joint compartment. As this broad adhesion is frequently formed at the anterior boundaries of the upper joint compartment, distinguishing the real capsule from this structure is not easy.

Grade 3 is defined as a band-like adhesion.

Grade 4 is defined as an extensive adhesion

Articular process Small flat projections on either side of a vertebra incorporating the articular surface.

Articulation The place where two or more bones unite; the active or passive progress of moving a joint through its allowed physiological range of motion; sometimes called 'joint mobilisation'.

AS Anterior-superior.

Asymmetrical stance One foot in front of the other.

Atlantoaxial joint A joint between the 1st and 2nd cervical vertebrae.

Atlanto-occipital joint A synovial joint between the occiput and the 1st cervical vertebra.

Atlas The 1st cervical vertebra.

Axial skeleton The part of the skeleton that consists of the bones of the head and trunk.

Axis The 2nd cervical vertebra.

Baroreflex sensitivity The baroreflex is the fastest mechanism to regulate acute blood pressure changes via controlling heart rate, contractility and peripheral resistance. The baroreflex or baroreceptor sensitivity (BRS) index is a measurement to quantify how much control the baroreflex has on the heart rate.

Biaxial joint A joint in which the rounded surface of an oval bone fits within a cup-shaped socket on the other bone, allowing movements in two planes.

Bifid Bifid means that the spinous process is divided into two clefts.

Bilateral Involving two or both sides.

Brevis Brief or short.

Buckled motion segments Dysfunction of the vertebrae generally accompanying more than one direction.

Bursa A fluid-filled sac that serves to reduce friction between a bone and the surrounding soft tissue.

Caudal Towards the tail/inferiorly.

Cavitation Refers to the formation and activity of gaseous bubbles (or cavities) within the synovial fluid of a joint.

Central motor excitability A transient but significant facilitation of change in motor neuron pool excitability.

Central sensitisation A condition of the nervous system that is associated with the development and maintenance of chronic pain. When central sensitisation occurs, the nervous system goes through a process called wind-up and gets regulated in a persistent state of high reactivity.

Cervical (C) Neck.

Circumduction The active or passive movement of a limb in a circular fashion (e.g., the circular motion of the ball-and-socket joint).

Coccyx Tip or end of the tailbone.

Collagen The main structural protein of connective tissue fibres.

Condyle The rounded articular prominence at the end of a bone.

Contact point The part of the patient's body where the therapist places the applicator.

Contraction A process in which muscle tension is increased, with or without change in overall length.

Contra-lateral On the opposite side.

Coronal/frontal Plane dividing the body into anterior and posterior parts by passing through it longitudinally from one side to the other.

Coronal axis A horizontal line extending from left to right. Flexion and extension movements usually occur around this axis.

Crack An audible sound that signifies a successful application of a manipulative procedure.

Cranial Towards the head/superiorly.

Deltoid muscle Thick, triangular-shaped muscle covering the shoulder.

Deviation Movement of the joint either laterally or medially from the anatomical midline.

Distal Further from the centre or the point of origin.

Distraction Force acting along a perpendicular to longitudinal axis to draw the structures apart.

Dorsum Back of the hand or top surface of the foot.

Epicondyle A rounded eminence above the condyle of a long bone.

Erector spinae muscles The erector spinae muscles are a group of long muscles that originate near the sacrum and extend vertically up the length of the back. The erector spinae muscles lie on each side of the vertebral column and extend alongside the lumbar, thoracic and cervical sections of the spine.

Eversion Foot-related movement in a lateral direction.

Extension Backward motion in a sagittal plane about a transverse axis. Straightening of a spinal curve (exception: cervical and lumbar spines) or internal angle.

Fascia The soft tissue component of the connective tissue system extending over the whole body just below the skin.

Fibrous joint A joint connected by fibrous connective tissue.

Flexion Bending movement that decreases a spinal curve (exception: thoracic spine) and internal angle.

Frontal plane A vertical plane through the longitudinal axis, dividing the body into anterior and posterior parts.

Gapping Medial and lateral – opening one side of a joint.

High-velocity, low-amplitude (HVLA) thrust There are many types of HVLA manipulation approaches, which can be defined as a passive manual therapeutic manoeuvre during which a synovial joint is carried beyond the normal physiological range of movement (in the direction of the restriction) without exceeding the boundaries of anatomical integrity.

Hoffmann reflex (H-reflex) responses The H-reflex (or Hoffmann's reflex) is a reflectory reaction of muscles after electrical stimulation of sensory fibres (Ia afferents stemming from muscle spindles) in their innervating nerves.

Hypertonicity A condition of unusually high muscle tension.

Hypoalgesia Decreased sensitivity to pain.

Hypothenar eminence The medial side of the hand palmar surface heel.

Impulse A sudden forceful push or driving force.

Inferior Bottom.

IM Inferior-medial.

Inhibition Soft-tissue technique: a local sustained force that is applied to a specific joint.

IS Inferior-superior.

Insertion The site of attachment of a muscle to the part to be moved.

Inversion Foot-related movement in a medial direction.

Ipsilateral On the same side.

Lateral Further away from the midline.

Lateral flexion Movement in a coronal (frontal) plane about an anterior-posterior axis. Also called side-bending.

Lower extremity Thigh, leg and foot.

LSP Lumbar spine.

Lumbar Lower back.

Manipulation A type of manual therapy in which a thrust is applied to the patient in order to produce mechanical responses.

MCP Metacarpal phalangeal joint.

Mechanoreceptor A sensory receptor that responds to mechanical stimuli.

Mechanosensitive Sensitive to mechanical stimuli such as pressure from a mechanosensitive ion channel.

Medial Closer to the midline.

Meniscoid Intercapsular synovial fold formed either in the embryo or as a result of trauma to the joint.

Mobilisation *See* **Articulation**.

Motor neurone activity A neuron that passes from the central nervous system or a ganglion toward or to a muscle and conducts a nerve impulse that causes movement.

Muscle-reflexogenic responses A monosynaptic reflex that provides automatic regulation of skeletal muscle length. When a muscle lengthens, the muscle spindle is stretched and its nerve activity increases. This increases alpha motor neuron activity, causing the muscle fibres to contract and thus resist the stretching.

Musculature The muscular system of a body or region of the body.

Nerve A group of long, thin fibres that transmits sensory or motor information to the brain.

Nociceptor Sensory receptor (neuron) that sends signals to cause the perception of pain in response to potentially damaging stimuli.

Nociception The sensation of pain due to neural processing of a harmful stimulus.

Occiput (O) The back of the head or skull.

Orthopaedics A branch of medicine that deals with the diagnosis and treatment of musculoskeletal diseases.

Osteopathy A branch of manual therapy that addresses the abnormalities of structure and function to aid the body's self-healing, self-regulating mechanisms.

Osteoporosis Atrophy of bone tissue, resulting from hormonal changes or lack of calcium or vitamin D.

Palmar Palm surface of the hand.

Paraesthesia Pins and needles sensation.

Paraspinal muscles Muscles that are adjacent to the vertebral column.

Passive motion Movement made by the therapist while the patient is relaxed or passive.

Patient Individual receiving treatment.

Pedicles The pedicle is a stub of bone that connects the lamina to the vertebral body to form the vertebral arch. Two short, stout processes extend from the sides of the vertebral body and join with broad flat plates of bone (laminae) to form a hollow archway that protects the spinal cord.

Plantar Sole surface of the foot.

Posterior Back.

PA Posterior-anterior.

PI Posterior-inferior.

PIP Proximal interphalangeal joint.

Pronation Applied to the hand, an act of turning the palmar surface/medial rotation. Applied to the foot, a combination of abduction or eversion in the tarsal or metatarsal joints.

Proximal Situated nearer to the origin of a point of attachment.

Quadriceps The large group of muscle at the front of the thigh that includes four distinct parts.

Receptor A structure on the cell surface that receives stimuli.

Reinforce Applying extra pressure in order to focus specifically on or protect another part of the body by placing the applicator.

Reflexogenic Causing a reflex effect.

Rotation Movement about an axis – internal, external or medial, lateral.

Sacroiliac joints (SIJ) Joints between the sacrum and the ilia.

Sacrum Tailbone between the two halves of the pelvis.

Sagittal Plane dividing the body into left and right portions by passing through it longitudinally, from the front to the back.

SC joint Sternoclavicular joint.

Shearing Action or force inclining to lead to two adjoining parts of an articulation to slide in the direction of their plane of contact relative to each other.

Side-bending *See* **Lateral flexion**.

Soft tissue Tissue other than bone or joint.

Somato-autonomic responses A somato-autonomic reflex is elicited by stimulation of somatic tissue (strictly speaking, tissue of the musculoskeletal system and the dermis of the skin), and manifesting as an alteration in autonomic nervous system function.

Somato-humoral pathways Refers to pathways involving bodily humors such as hormones or immune responses that involves secretion of antibodies by B cells.

Somatosensory processing The somatosensory system is the part of the sensory system concerned with the conscious perception of touch, pressure, pain, temperature, position, movement, and vibration, which arise from the muscles, joints, skin, and fascia.

Sprain Tearing or stretching of ligaments and/or tendons of a joint.

Superficial Nearer to the body surface.

Superior Top.

SI Superior-inferior.

SP Spinous process.

Supination Applied to the hand: turning the palm forward or upward by lateral external rotation of the forearm; applied to the foot: applying adduction and inversion movement to the medial margin of the foot.

Supraspinal Supraspinal means above the spine and may refer to above the spinal cord and vertebral column: brain.

Symmetrical stance Feet are side by side.

Sympathetic activity A part of the nervous system that serves to accelerate the heart rate, constrict blood vessels and raise blood pressure.

Sympatheticexcitatory response A part of the nervous system that serves to accelerate the heart rate, constrict blood vessels, and raise blood pressure.

Symphyses A fusion between two articulating bones separated by a pad of fibrocartilage.

Syndesmosis An immovable joint bound by interosseous ligaments.

Synovial A type of joint that contains a lubricating substance (synovial fluid) and is lined with a thick flexible membrane.

Synovial fold A pleat of the synovial membrane located on the inner surface of the joint capsule.

Tactile Pertaining to the sense of touch.

Temporomandibular joint (TMJ) manipulation techniques These are manipulation techniques applied to the temporal and mandibular bones which create the TMJ.

Thenar eminence The lateral side of the hand palmar surface heel.

Thoracic (T)/Dorsal (D) Mid and upper back.

Thorax The region of the body located between the neck and the abdomen.

Thrust An external force applied during manipulation.

Traction Force acting along a longitudinal axis in order to draw the structures apart.

Translation Motion along an axis.

Transverse Plane dividing the body into upper and lower portions by passing perpendicular to sagittal and frontal planes horizontally through the body.

Trunk The part of the human body extending from the neck to pelvic region.

TVP Transverse process.

Uncovertebral joints Uncovertebral joints, also known as Luschka's joints, are formed between uncinate process or 'uncus' below and uncovertebral articulation above. They are located in the cervical region of the vertebral column between C3 and C7.

Unilateral Pertaining to one side of a structure.

Upper extremity Arm, forearm and hand.

Vascular Relating to vessels or ducts that convey blood and lymph.

Ventral *See* **Anterior**.

Visceral Relating to the viscera or the internal organs of the body.

Zygapophysial joints A set of synovial joints formed joining the superior and inferior articular processes.

Subject Index

Author Index